# SRB's Atlas of
# Tissue Approximation with Suturing and Knotting

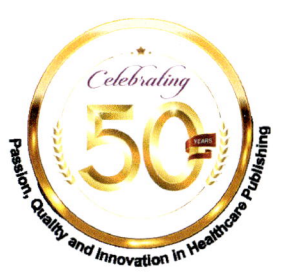

# Video Contents

*There are two videos along with this Atlas, available on eMedicine360.com*

### Suturing Video 1: Suturing Techniques Demonstrated on Models, Foams and Bars (1 Hour 3 Minutes)

- Instruments Holding
- Simple Interrupted Suture
- Simple Continuous Suture
- Continuous Interlocking Suture (Ford Suture)
- Continuous Blanket Suture
- Vertical Mattress Suture (Far-Far and Near-Near)
- Vertical Mattress Suture (Near-Near and Far-Far)
- Vertical Pulley Suture (Far-Near and Near-Far)
- All-Gower Suture
- Horizontal Mattress Suture
- Granny Knot
- Instrument Granny Knot
- Reef Knot
- Instrument Reef Knot
- Surgeon's Knot
- Instrument Surgeon's Knot
- Aberdeen Knot
- Single Hand Knot
- Single Hand Reef Knot
- Single Hand Surgeon's Knot
- Two Hand Reef Knot
- Two Hand Surgeon's Knot
- Suture Removal

### Suturing Video 2: Live Demonstration of Suturing Techniques (32 Minutes)

- Instrument and Suture Handling
- Simple Interrupted Suture
- Interrupted Vertical Mattress Suture
- Vertical Mattress Suture (Far-Far and Near-Near)
- Vertical Mattress Suture (Near-Near and Far-Far)
- All-Gower Suturing
- Continuous Peritoneal Closure
- Aberdeen Knot
- Subcutaneous Suturing
- Subcuticular Suturing
- Dermal Approximation
- Drain Fixation
- Clip Removal

# SRB's Atlas of Tissue Approximation with Suturing and Knotting

**Sriram Bhat M** MS (General Surgery)
Professor and Head
Department of Surgery
Kasturba Medical College, Mangalore
Mangaluru, Karnataka, India
Honorary Surgeon
Government District Wenlock Hospital
Mangaluru, Karnataka, India

*Foreword*
K Jayarama Shenoy

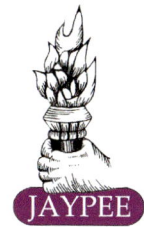

**JAYPEE BROTHERS MEDICAL PUBLISHERS**
*The Health Sciences Publisher*
New Delhi | London

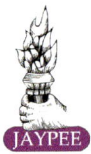

**Jaypee Brothers Medical Publishers (P) Ltd.**

**Headquarters**
Jaypee Brothers Medical Publishers (P) Ltd
4838/24, Ansari Road, Daryaganj
New Delhi 110 002, India
Phone: +91-11-43574357
Fax: +91-11-43574314
Email: jaypee@jaypeebrothers.com

**Overseas Office**
J.P. Medical Ltd
83 Victoria Street, London
SW1H 0HW (UK)
Phone: +44 20 3170 8910
Fax: +44 (0)20 3008 6180
Email: info@jpmedpub.com

Website: www.jaypeebrothers.com
Website: www.jaypeedigital.com

© 2021, Jaypee Brothers Medical Publishers

The views and opinions expressed in this book are solely those of the original contributor(s)/author(s) and do not necessarily represent those of editor(s) of the book.

All rights reserved. No part of this publication may be reproduced, stored or transmitted in any form or by any means, electronic, mechanical, photocopying, recording or otherwise, without the prior permission in writing of the publishers.

All brand names and product names used in this book are trade names, service marks, trademarks or registered trademarks of their respective owners. The publisher is not associated with any product or vendor mentioned in this book.

Medical knowledge and practice change constantly. This book is designed to provide accurate, authoritative information about the subject matter in question. However, readers are advised to check the most current information available on procedures included and check information from the manufacturer of each product to be administered, to verify the recommended dose, formula, method and duration of administration, adverse effects and contraindications. It is the responsibility of the practitioner to take all appropriate safety precautions. Neither the publisher nor the author(s)/editor(s) assume any liability for any injury and/or damage to persons or property arising from or related to use of material in this book.

This book is sold on the understanding that the publisher is not engaged in providing professional medical services. If such advice or services are required, the services of a competent medical professional should be sought.

Every effort has been made where necessary to contact holders of copyright to obtain permission to reproduce copyright material. If any have been inadvertently overlooked, the publisher will be pleased to make the necessary arrangements at the first opportunity. The **CD/DVD-ROM** (if any) provided in the sealed envelope with this book is complimentary and free of cost. **Not meant for sale**.

**Inquiries for bulk sales may be solicited at:** jaypee@jaypeebrothers.com

*SRB's Atlas of Tissue Approximation with Suturing and Knotting*

*First Edition:* **2021**

ISBN: 978-81-947090-0-8

*Printed at Replika Press Pvt. Ltd.*

# Dedicated to

*My Late Grand Parents*

**(Late) Mrs and Mr Rama Bhat**  **(Late) Mrs and Mr Krishna Bhat**

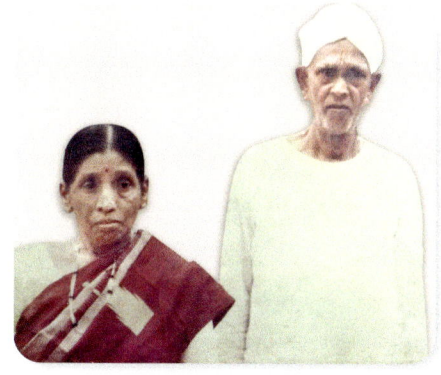
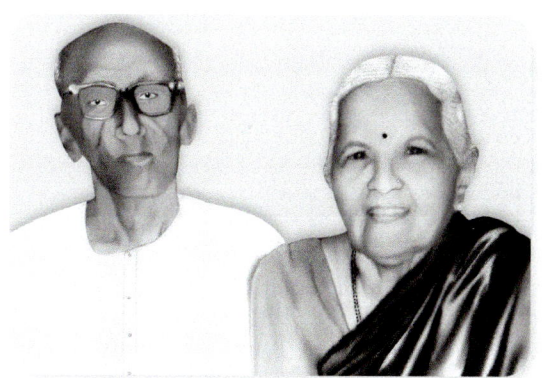

*AND*
*Also to all COVID patients*
*who succumbed globally worldwide*
*and to COVID Warriors*
*who selflessly worked to save the mankind from pandemic.*

# Foreword

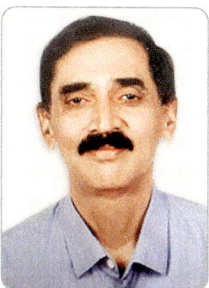

As Dr Sriram Bhat M, Professor and Head, Department of Surgery, Kasturba Medical College, Mangalore, is presenting his new major book on surgical education entitled *SRB's Atlas of Tissue Approximation with Suturing and Knotting*, I am honored and proud to write the foreword, honored—to associate with the good work of Dr Sriram Bhat M, an acclaimed surgical teacher in and outside the country and proud—to have played a small role in Dr Sriram's early years as his teacher and mentor.

Dr Sriram has chosen an important part of surgical science, that makes an art too, that is aimed at providing clarity to the surgical residents and students on the tissue approximation and knotting, an integral part of surgery, a science and art involving application of appropriate knowledge and skill to achieve healing of the wounds.

The book has seven chapters, divided into different levels and aspects of tissue approximation, starting from the historic evolution of the scientific art, knowledge-based conceptualization leading to the actual performance of the art in its various forms, conventional and modern, apt to the contemporary practice of surgery, including the suturing and knotting techniques in minimally invasive surgery. The chapters are rich with illustrations, diagrams and photographs to enrich one's experience of "virtually being there". I am also glad that Dr Sriram Bhat M has shared videos with the book for helping the students learn faster and better.

The students and practitioners of surgery will find this book very useful as a guide.

My good wishes to Dr Sriram Bhat M.

**K Jayarama Shenoy**
Senior Surgical Consultant, Mangaluru
Former Head
Kasturba Medical College, Mangalore
Mangaluru, Karnataka, India

# Preface

After writing surgical books such as manual, operative surgery, clinical books, I felt still incomplete in my work as I thought basic essentiality for a skilled surgeon other than fine anatomical dissection is perfect tissue approximation at different situations in different tissues. My teachers used to say, "*Use the suture needle of suitable shape and size; use the suture material that is of suitable type and size for the tissues being sutured*". "*Approximate and not strangulate the tissue*" is the common dictum, we are taught.

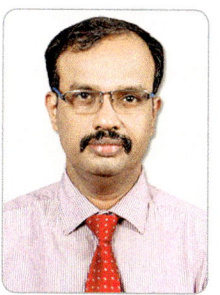

I slowly started formulating my ideas into a book but took more time to establish compared to my earlier books, probably because once I started writing the manuscript, I understood that this subject is more complex, complicated and confusing rather than simple. There are seven chapters in the book. Initial chapters highlight the history, instruments and basics; eventual chapters discuss the proper method of suturing and knotting techniques with principles. Adequate illustrations and photos are also the better part of the book. A brief but adequate highlight on laparoscopic suturing is also dealt with. This book is handy but adequately informative and could become an essential commodity to all surgical trainees as well as practicing surgeons including specialties as this basis is essential pillar of surgical skill in operative surgery. I thank my beloved teacher, Professor K Jayarama Shenoy, Senior Surgical Consultant, Mangaluru, and Former Head, Department of Surgery, Kasturba Medical College, Mangalore, for writing foreword to this book. By being with him as junior consultant during my initial career of profession and later also, I could acquire part of his immense knowledge on surgical anatomy, clinical principles and skill too.

I thank all my colleagues, postgraduates and publisher for helping me to bringing this book. Hope readers will enjoy and understand the book well. I welcome healthy constructive criticism to improve the book in subsequent editions.

**Sriram Bhat M** MS (General surgery)
Professor and Head
Department of Surgery
Kasturba Medical College, Mangalore
Mangaluru, Karnataka, India
Honorary Surgeon
Government District Wenlock Hospital
Mangaluru, Karnataka, India
*meera_sriram2003@yahoo.com*

# Acknowledgments

It is impossible to bring out a book without help of so many.

I thank our Chancellor, Dr Ramdas M Pai; Pro-Chancellor Dr HS Ballal; Vice Chancellor of Manipal Academy of Higher Education (MAHE), Lt Gen Dr MD Venkatesh; Pro-Vice Chancellor Dr Poornima Baliga and Dr Dilip G Naik.

I thank our beloved Dean, Dr Venkatraya Prabhu for his support and help throughout my carrier.

I thank Additional Dean, Dr Alfred Augustine, Vice Deans, Dr Unnikrishnan and Dr Nuthan Kamath for their affectionate help.

I thank my beloved teacher, Professor Jayarama Shenoy for writing foreword to this book. He is my teacher from whom I have learnt surgical skills both basic and advanced; surgical principles and ethics in surgery. A devoted teacher and surgeon, students across the world adore him for his teaching and principles.

I thank all my colleagues in Department of Surgery, Kasturba Medical College, Mangalore.

I thank faculties of Department of Dental Surgery, Mangalore, for their kind help always. I thank Dr Stanley Mathew, Professor and Head, Department of Surgery, Kasturba Medical College, Manipal and all his faculties.

I would like to remember all my teachers by whom what I am today. I always seek their blessings with humbleness.

My special thanks to DMO, Government Wenlock Hospital, Mangaluru, Dr Sadashiva Shanbogue and all medical officers and also other staffs. It is always important to remember my beloved patients who are the inspiration and resource for all my professional and academic works. Earlier DMO, Dr Rajeshwari Madam also should be remembered for her all encouragements towards my work.

I thank my friend, Dr Ganapathi, Anesthesiologist and Director, Mangala Hospital and Mangala Kidney Foundation, Kadri, Mangaluru, for his constant unconditional help in all my endeavors.

I also thank my beloved friend, a dedicated Urologist, Dr Ashok Pandit, Yenepoya Specialty Hospital, Mangaluru who taught me every basic skills of surgery selflessly in last 30 years. I owe him a lot.

I greatly acknowledge Dr Ganesh MK; Laparoscopic Surgeon, Father Muller's Hospital and Medical College, Mangaluru, Karnataka, and Dr Keshavprasad, Associate Professor, Kasturba Medical College, Mangalore, for helping me in getting quality photographs for the book.

I thank all my undergraduate and postgraduate students and interns for their help in getting photographs and doing illustrations.

Three people I need thank specifically are Dr Bhargav Vyas AN, Assistant Professor, Department of Surgery, Kasturba Medical College, Mangalore, Mangaluru; Dr Balodi Divya Maheshbhai and Dr Akshay Kantha, surgical postgraduates; they have helped me with real affection in all editing, collecting photographs, taking videos. I really owe them a lot.

I thank and appreciate Shri Jitendar P Vij (Group Chairman) whom I consider as mentor for writing books. His encouragement and motivation is a driving force for me.

I thank Mr Ankit Vij (Managing Director), Mr MS Mani (Group President), Ms Chetna Malhotra Vohra (Associate Director–Content Strategy), Ms Pooja Bhandari (Production Head), Dr Savleen Kaur (Development Editor) and all staff of M/s Jaypee Brothers Medical Publishers (P) Ltd, New Delhi, India, for doing appreciable work in their respective field of printing and publishing. Also, my appreciation to working team in M/s Jaypee Brothers Medical Publishers (Bengaluru and Mangaluru Branches), for their timely help.

# Contents

1. Basis of Suturing ............................................................................................................................. 1

2. Instruments for Suturing ............................................................................................................. 3

3. Suture Materials and Needles ................................................................................................... 13

4. Principles of Suturing ................................................................................................................. 27

5. Surgical Knot Tying ..................................................................................................................... 35

6. Skin and Soft Tissue Suturing ................................................................................................... 46

7. Laparoscopic Suturing and Knotting ...................................................................................... 69

*Index* .................................................................................................................................................. *89*

# CHAPTER 1: Basis of Suturing

*No operation should be carried out unless absolutely necessary ... nor should a surgeon operate unless he would undergo the same operation himself in similar circumstances, ... The Knife Man: The Extraordinary Life and Times of John Hunter, Father of Scientific Surgery.*

## INTRODUCTION

Surgery basically is a *science* with *art* and *principle. The two essential parts of the surgery* are—*surgical dissection* which needs clear idea about the biology of disease, surgical anatomy of the area and clear technical approaches of dissection; and *suturing and knotting* which is the basic essential entity needed after surgical dissection which facilitates the accurate and secure tissue approximation, minimizes the bleeding and infection, supports the wound, apposes the skin/tissue edge. "Suture" word is derived from the *Latin* word—*sutura*. Suture means to "sew" or "seam". In surgery, suture is the act of sewing or bringing tissue together and holding them in apposition until healing has taken place.

*Dissection is the art of executing the correction of the pathology whereas suturing is the re-establishing the anatomy allowing the best possible physiological and physical outcome.* In open surgery, technique is done with direct vision with surgeon's hand in line with visual axis and so execution of suturing and knotting is done in semi-automatic fashion.

*Surgical suture* is basically a device used to keep the body tissues together after an injury or break either by trauma or after surgical operation. A needle with attached suture material of needed size is passed through the tissues and secured afterwards with a surgical knot. A suture is a strand of material used to ligate blood vessels and to approximate tissues together.

*Ambroise Pare* (1520–1590), a French surgeon, introduced the concept of gentleness in wound care which reduces the inflammation and promotes healing; he said, *"I dress the wound; God heals them".* He used sticking strips of plaster to approximate wounds of the face **(Figs. 1A and B)**.

Perhaps the world's oldest suture was placed by an embalmer on the body of a 21st dynasty mummy about 1100 BC. Eyed needles were in use during ancient times (4000 BC). African tribes used to ligate the vessels using tendons and vegetations. A South American method of wound closure used large black ants which were made to bite the wound edges together and the ant's body is then twisted off leaving the head in place. East African tribes ligated blood vessels with tendons and closed wounds with acacia thorns.

Surgical sutures were used as early as 3000 BC by ancient Egypt. Egyptians (1600 BC) were using linen strips coated with honey and flour as suture materials. Sushrutha from India in 500 BC had written detailed notes on surgical sutures and wound suturing. He described round bodied, triangular, curved, straight needles in his book. Sutures used were from plants like flax (blue-colored plant), cannabis (hemp), bark fiber (cotton), and hairs.

Sometime around 30 AD, a medical encyclopedia was written by a Roman named Aurelius Cornelius Celsus. His work, De Re Medicina, tells the reader that sutures should be "soft, and not over twisted, so that they may be more easy on the part." He is also credited with first substantiated mention of ligating by recommending it as a secondary means of stopping a hemorrhage. Galen from Rome (150 AD) described gut sutures **(Fig. 2)**. In 10th century, catgut was manufactured using sheep or cattle intestines. The origin of the word "catgut" is not sure; probably either it was derived from cattle gut or it was easily available in ancient times from musicians

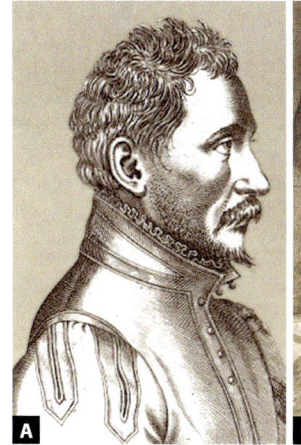
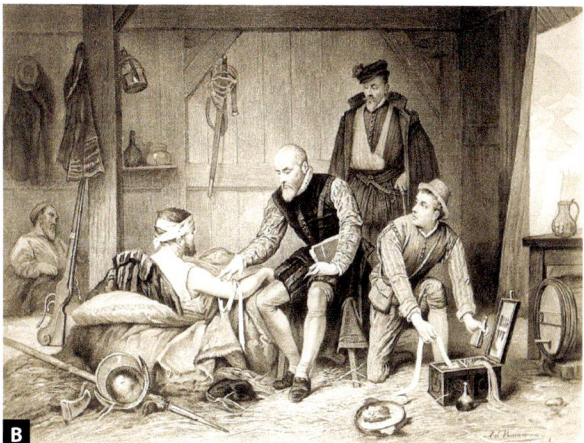

**Figs. 1A and B:** Ambroise Pare.

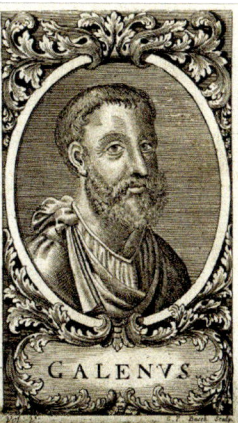

**Fig. 2:** Claudius Galen.

Claudius Galen is a Roman physician and philosopher of Greek origin. He earned a reputation as a practitioner and a public demonstrator of anatomy as he performed extensive dissections and vivisections on animals. He described many formulae containing plants and animal drugs, which he compiled this knowledge in 20 books called as Galenical works. His theories dominated and influenced the medical science for well over a million.

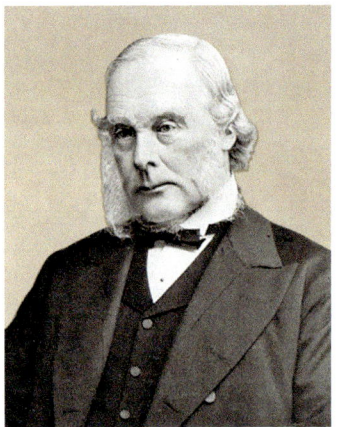

**Fig. 3:** Joseph Lister.
Sir Joseph Lister—British surgeon and pioneer of antiseptic surgery; he is being called as "Father of Modern Surgery".

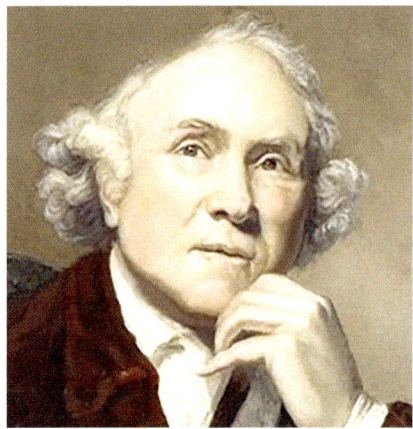

**Fig. 4:** John Hunter.
John Hunter (13th Feb 1728–16th Oct 1793) Scottish anatomist, surgeon and pathologist who was an early advocate of investigation and experimentation, and a founder of pathological anatomy in England. He made many important studies in comparative aspects of biology, anatomy, physiology, and pathology.

(Kit is an ancient musical instrument, looked-like violin where catgut/kitgut was used as string).

Rhazes of Arabia was credited for first employing "kitgut" to suture abdominal wounds in 900 AD. The Arabic word "kit" means a dancing master's fiddle the musical strings in which "kit string" were made up of sheep intestines. Over the years, "kit" was confused with kitten or cat, and the misuse of the term was propagated. Albucasis (AD 936) used double sutures. Andreas Vesalius first advocated the suture of all fresh wounds as well as severed tendon and nerves.

Joseph Lister (1827-1912) discovered that bacteria present in suture strands caused wound infection **(Fig. 3)**. He disinfected sutures with carbolic acid. He made sterile sutures possible to bury it in clean wounds without infection.

First monofilament suture, pig's bristle is used by Avicenna. John Hunter used interrupted sutures, sticking plasters **(Fig. 4)**. He postulated uses of absorbable sutures which get dissolved and disappear after its function is over. Joseph Lister started sterilization of all suture materials using carbolic acid in 1860. Joseph Lister is the founder of the principles of antisepsis and asepsis. He started usage of ligatures for aneurysms; he identified the principles of absorption of catgut. George Merson, pharmacist from Edinburgh during World War I, started eyeless needled suture materials calling them as "Mersutures". After 1930, synthetic suture materials such as polyvinyl alcohol, polyesters, and polyglycolic acid (1960) were discovered. In 1970, polyglycolic acid became popular synthetic suture material. Halsted **(Fig. 5)** popularized the silk suture material.

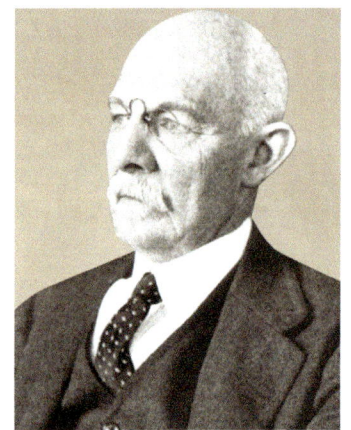

**Fig. 5:** William Stewart Halsted
William Stewart Halsted (1852–1922). He was from New York, America. A renowned surgeon, teacher who popularized residency training programme in surgery. Halsted hernia surgery, Halsted radical mastectomy, Halsted ligament (condensed clavipectoral fascia), Halsted mosquito forceps, Halsted apical axillary lymph node, Halsted mattress suture, use of surgical gloves are his other contributions. Halsted pioneered his principles (Halsted Principles) of control of bleeding, accurate anatomical dissection, complete sterility, exact approximation of tissue in wound closures without excessive tightness, and gentle handling of tissues.

## Fundamental Basis of Suturing

- Accurate and fine coating of the wound edges.
- Adequate wound support.
- Achieving the eversion of the wound edges as much as possible.
- Allowing the shift of the tension into the deeper part of the wound.
- Achieving minimal tension over the superficial part of the wound edge in the wound surface which will yield the most cosmetically acceptable scar.
- Achieving a functional and esthetically acceptable closure.
- Wound edges should be smooth and perpendicular to the surface.
- Integrity of the blood supply should not be compromised.

## Technical Basis of Suturing

- Proper selection of the needle type in relation to its curvature and size and also needle holder (driver).
- Selection of ideal size of the suture material.
- Right technique with optimal spacing.
- Optimum grip and stability with optimum precision.
- Attaining direct binocular vision with surgeon's hand in line with visual axis.
- Traumatic wounds more often need debridement and proper prior planning and alignment to achieve tension free suturing whereas surgical incisions/wounds are planned and clean and so easier to approximate.

*Surgery is an art with science;* suturing is the essential basis in tissue approximation. Since different tissues and different parts of the body have different dynamics, suturing type and material type and technique may differ in each situation; complex dynamic, science, and skill should be achieved by surgeon with repeated thinking and practice.

In *laparoscopic suturing*, the situation is different. Image is magnified and indirect; and so suturing and knotting technique will not be as easy and fluent as in open surgery. It needs cognitive and psychomotor skills for laparoscopic suturing; it needs necessary choreography and maneuvers to have a safe, effective tissue approximation.

Since laparoscopic surgery is equally gaining importance, along with technique of open surgery suturing, it is also discussed in detail in this book.

## TERMINOLOGIES

- Each 'needle bite' means needle passing through the single edge of the wound.
- 'Single large bite' means needle bite enters through the skin/tissue on one side and comes out of the opposite edge of the tissue (means both edges of the wound together) to proceed for knotting.
- 'Each throw' is a single half knot. Usually, three throws (three half knots) are used. In suture material-like polypropylene, five throws are used to avoid knot slippage.

# CHAPTER 2: Instruments for Suturing

*"Imagination is more important than knowledge. Knowledge is limited. Imagination encircles the world."*
–Albert Einstein

## INTRODUCTION

It is always essential to have proper idea about the instruments being used for suturing. Unless surgeon knows the details about the instruments, he may struggle while doing the suturing technique.

For simple suturing, basic suturing instruments are sufficient. For difficult suturing specialized sutures and instruments are needed like in laparoscopic suturing; or in fine suturing wherein loupes are used to achieve magnification.

Basic ergonomics, surgical anatomy, tissue alignment, precise movements at wrist and elbow; adequate length, curvature of the instruments are essential needs. Instrument should function as an extension of surgeon's hands.

*Basic instruments* **(Fig. 1)** *used are:*
- Needle driver (holder)
- Suture materials and needles
- Tissue forceps—toothed and non-toothed
- *Gauze:* Nonwoven gauze (it is better than woven gauze as its wicking property is excellent and it does not unravel) and mop
- Scalpel blade
- Hemostat
- Suture-cutting straight scissor
- Cautery

Instruments are held in two ways: *Better method* is by *finger-tip pressure* wherein thumb and ring fingers are placed in finger bows of the instrument. Precise fine-relaxed movements are essential for proper work-up of the instruments. Bizarre-hurried movements will not give precision. *Second method* of holding the instruments is tight *vise-like grip* using fist of the hand. It gives a good grip but precision may not be adequate. Surgical trainee to begin with prefers this method as he will think that grip is essential part in holding the instrument. Even though this method may be useful in some situations, it is ideal to use the method of finger-tip pressure and practice it for eventual smooth precise work. Middle finger of the surgeon is kept behind the handle and index finger is extended along the length of the handle. It is said that slow, definitive, precise, and nonrepetitive movements actually yield faster surgery than haphazard, frenzied, and rapid movements **(Fig. 2)**.

*Holding the instrument:* Finger-tip pressure (finger grip) is better to hold instruments than vise grip. But it is finally surgeon's choice and comfort.

Hemostasis is achieved using coagulation cautery. Dissection using coagulation cautery will be hemostatic but causes boiling of fat, more tissue trauma leading into wound infection. Ideally over coagulation of tissues during cautery dissection should be avoided.

Tissues are held using forceps by gentle maneuver. Skin and tough structures are held using toothed forceps; soft, smooth, delicate structures should be held using non-toothed forceps.

*Needle holder* should be held between thumb and ring fingers to achieve rotation movement using wrist (not pushing movement). Index and middle fingers are used to steady the handle. Needle is laced at the junction of proximal 2/3rd and distal 1/3rd of the distal jaws.

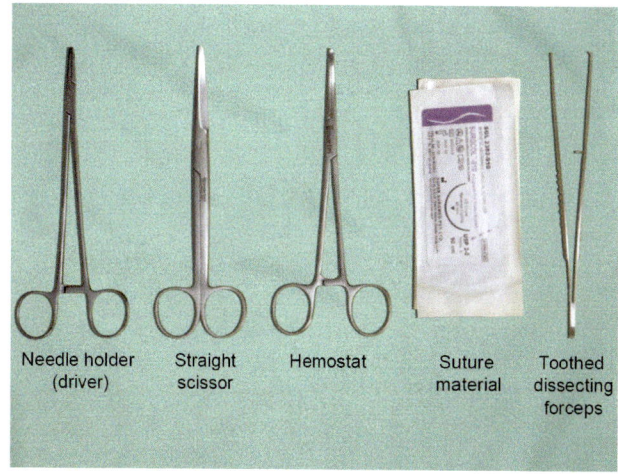

**Fig. 1:** Basic instruments required for suturing.

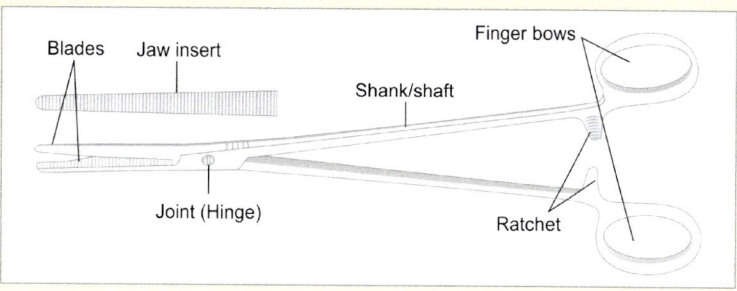

**Fig. 2:** Parts of a surgical instrument.

## NEEDLE HOLDER (NEEDLE DRIVER)

It is strong and sturdy instrument with long proximal blades and short distal blades (**Figs. 3A to C**). Ends are rounded distally with their flat inner surface to grasp the needle (**Figs. 4A and B**). Inner surface can be serrated or nonserrated (smooth jaw); (serrations when present are criss-cross typed); with a groove or without. Serrations add stability and optimum grip to the needle but may damage grasped suture while knotting. Ratio of length of handle (shank/shaft) to blade (jaw) is usually 4:1.

Different needle holders are available with different lengths and curvatures. Fine-needle holders are also available. There are especially designed needle holders for fine-suturing of vessels, and also especially in ophthalmology where microscopy is used for suturing and for this purpose needles are small and precision is important. *Webster-Halsey, Mayo Hegar, Baumgartner*—are different needle holders used (**Figs. 5 and 6**).

Needle is placed near the end of the needle holder usually at a point at the junction of proximal 2/3rd and distal 1/3rd to have optimal control and grip (**Fig. 7**). Needle is held near its swaged end or in the middle or toward the tip depending on the arc needed during tissue bite; which is finally assessed by the depth of the tissue and space available in the depth for easy maneuverability. After placing the needle, needle holder is closed firmly usually to its full extent with a single click. Needle should be held firmly to avoid slippage and inadvertent movements; usually ring finger and thumb are used to hold the needle holder. Palming position, grasping position, and holding with thenar prominence are different positions used (**Figs. 8 and 9**). Holding with fingers is the standard position, but depending on the need, the depth and type of tissues to be approximated, surgeon may change the holding. *Needle holder is usually (ideally) to be held by placing thumb and ring fingers into the finger bows and middle finger supports the bow and index finger supports the shank/shaft of the needle holder.*

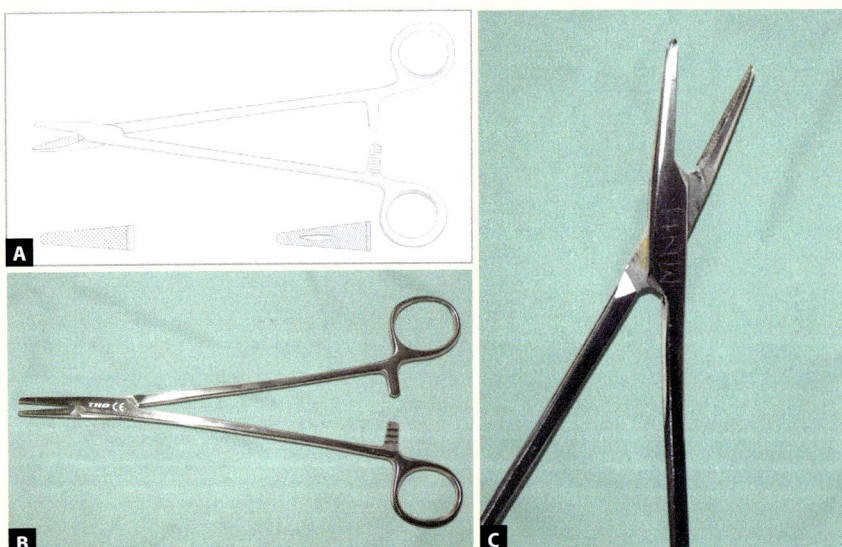

**Figs. 3A to C:** Parts of the needle holder.

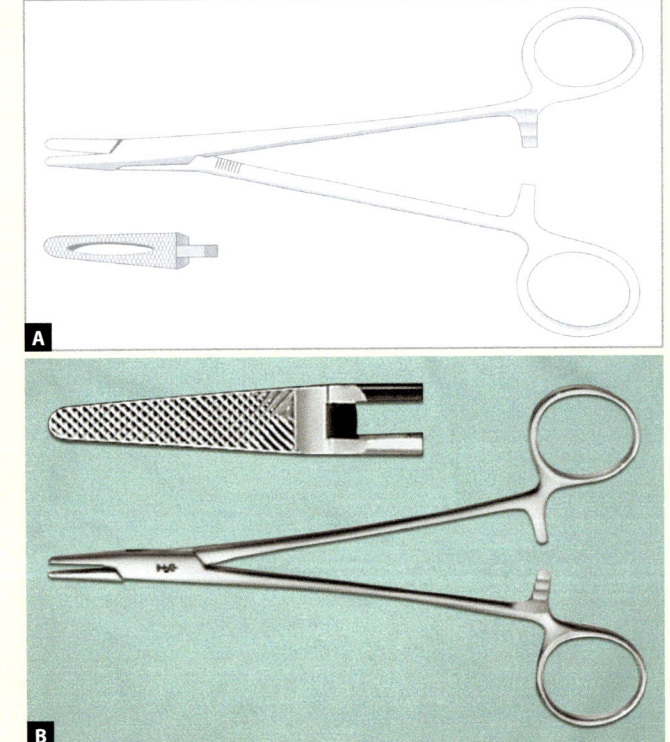

**Figs. 4A and B:** Needle holder—distal end.

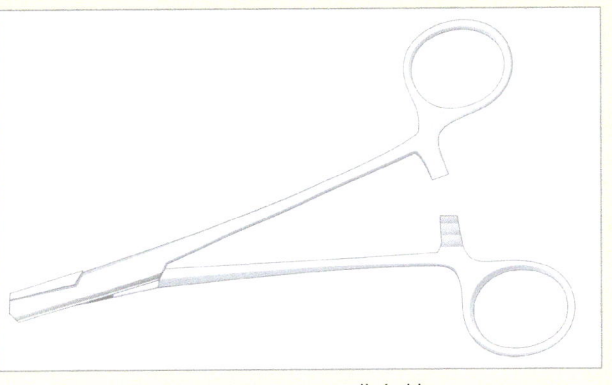

**Fig. 5:** Mayo Hegar needle holder.

## TISSUE FORCEPS (DISSECTING FORCEPS)

Tissue forceps are essential instrument in surgery; it is used to hold tissues while dissecting as well as approximating (**Figs 10A and B**). Different types and sized forceps are available. Usually, it is held like a pen. Fine forceps such as *Adson's forceps* are used in finer tissue apposition. *Bishop Harmon forceps* is used for delicate tissue apposition (**Figs. 11A and B**). Forceps may be toothed

Instruments for Suturing

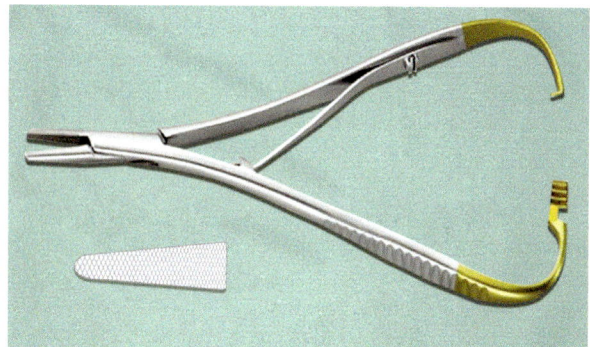

**Fig. 6:** Baumgartner specialized needle holder.

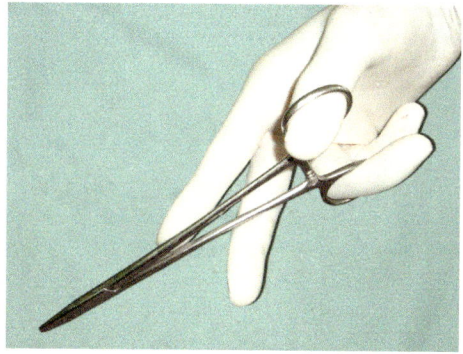

**Fig. 7:** Holding the needle holder properly and knowing its movement in rotational axis is important for proper suturing and knotting. It is the precise gentle rotation which is essential; not pushing flimsy movement. The needle holder is held with thumb and ring finger through the rings and with the index finger along the length of needle holder to provide stability and control.

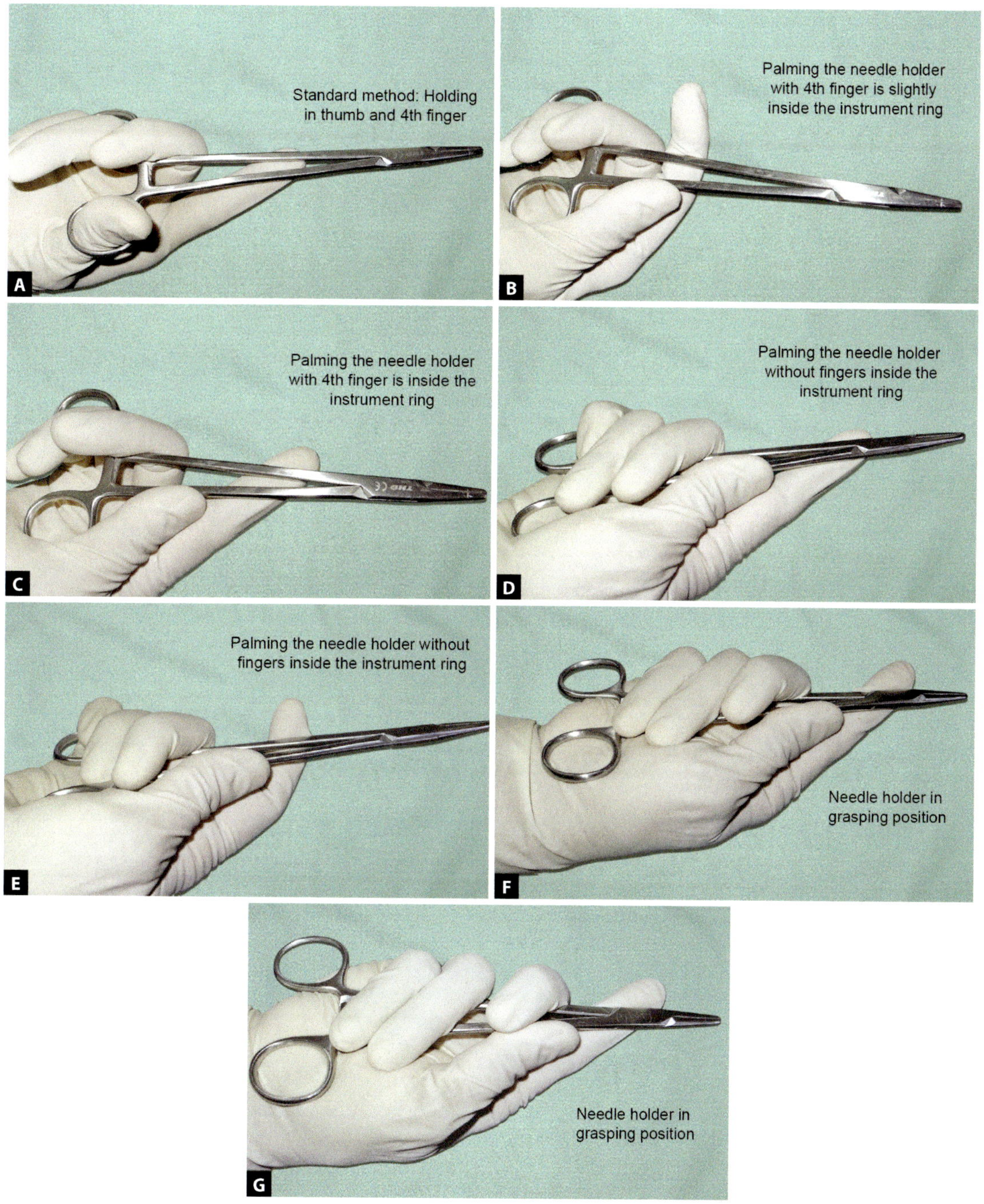

A — Standard method: Holding in thumb and 4th finger

B — Palming the needle holder with 4th finger is slightly inside the instrument ring

C — Palming the needle holder with 4th finger is inside the instrument ring

D — Palming the needle holder without fingers inside the instrument ring

E — Palming the needle holder without fingers inside the instrument ring

F — Needle holder in grasping position

G — Needle holder in grasping position

**Figs. 8A to G:** Different ways of holding the needle holder.

**Figs. 9A to D:** Placing the needle in needle holder.

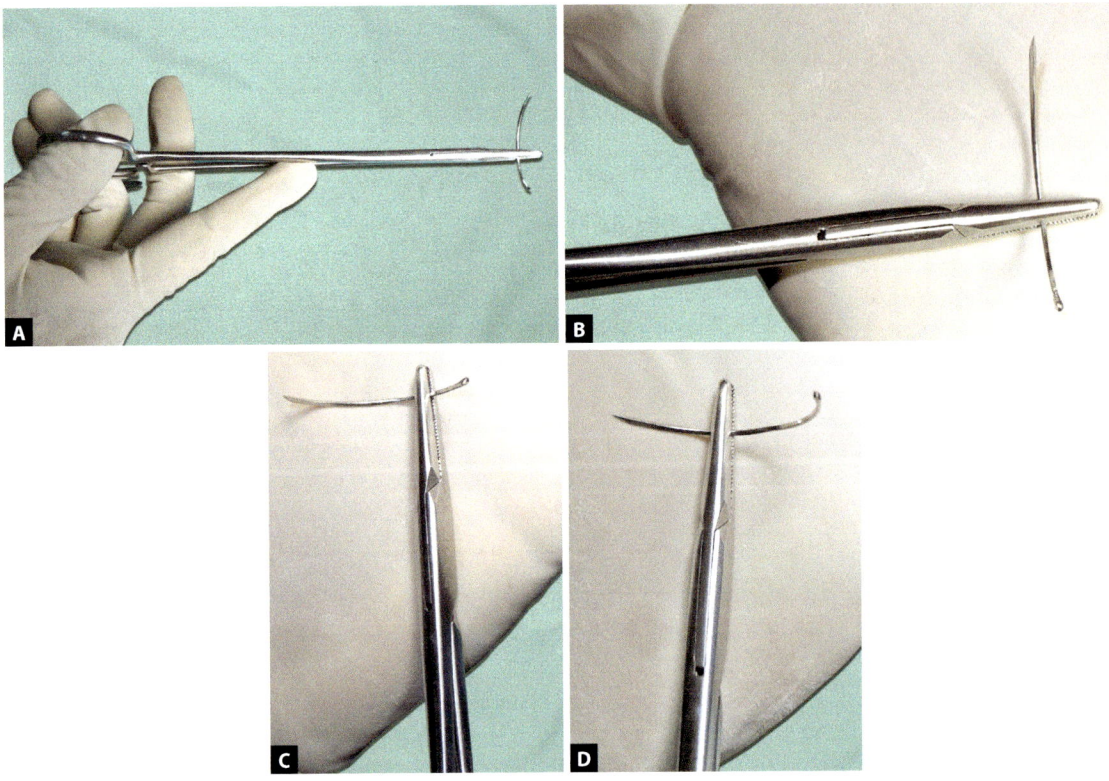

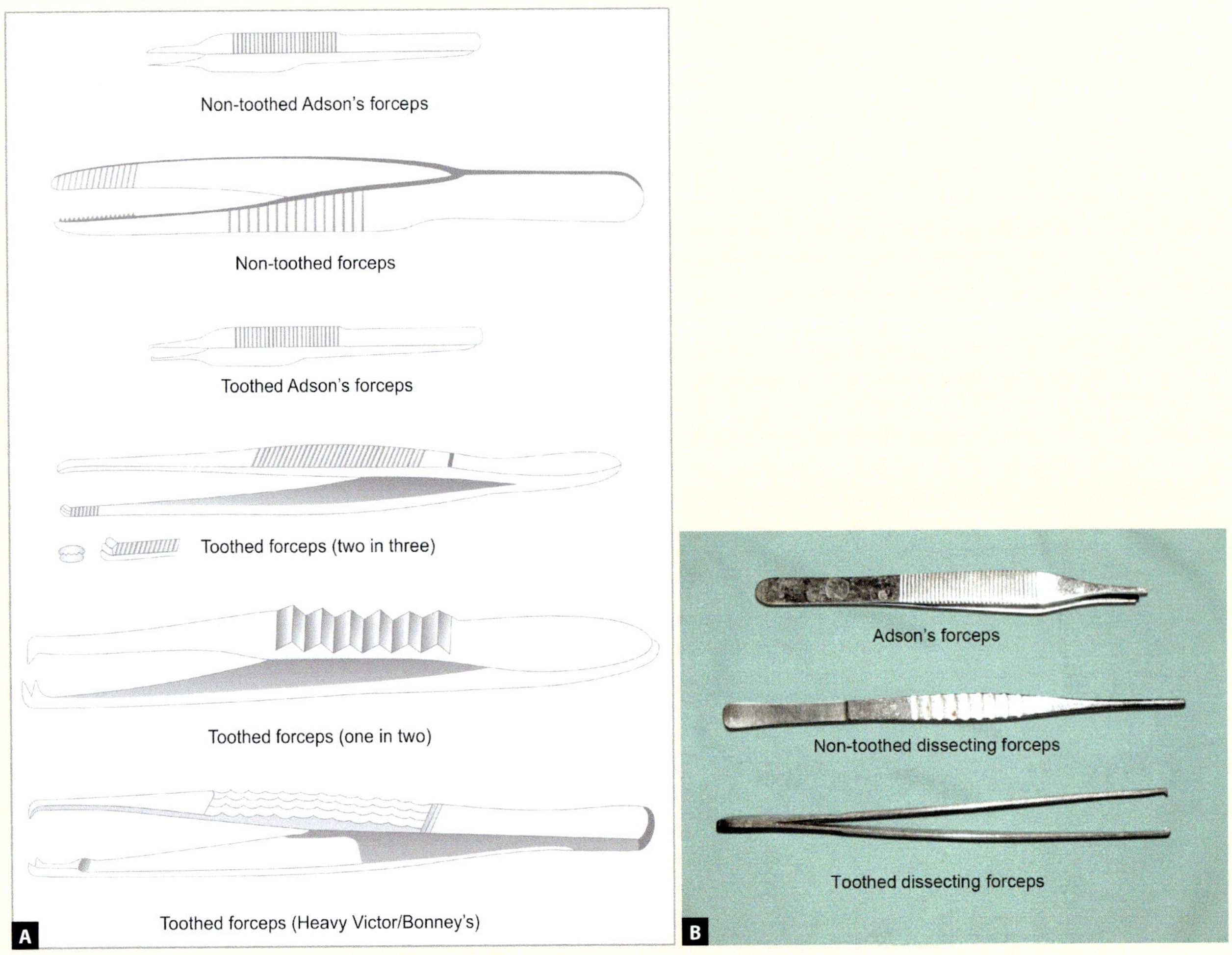

**Figs. 10A and B:** Dissecting forceps used in tissue approximation.

## Instruments for Suturing

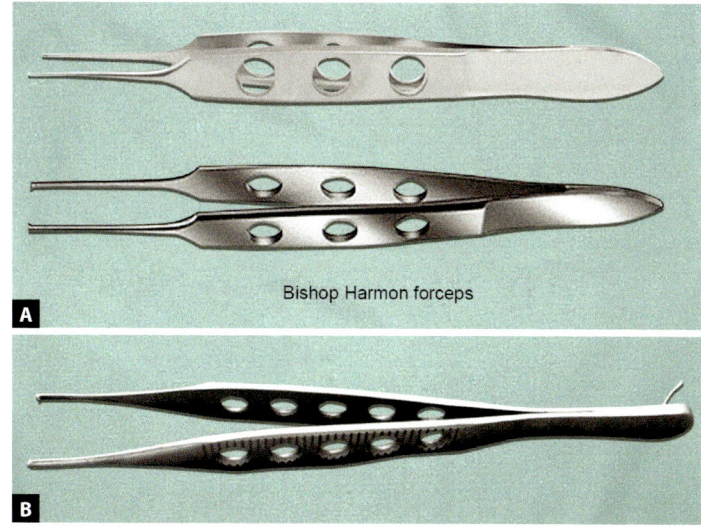

**Figs. 11A and B:** Bishop Harmon forceps—it is used in fine delicate tissue suturing.

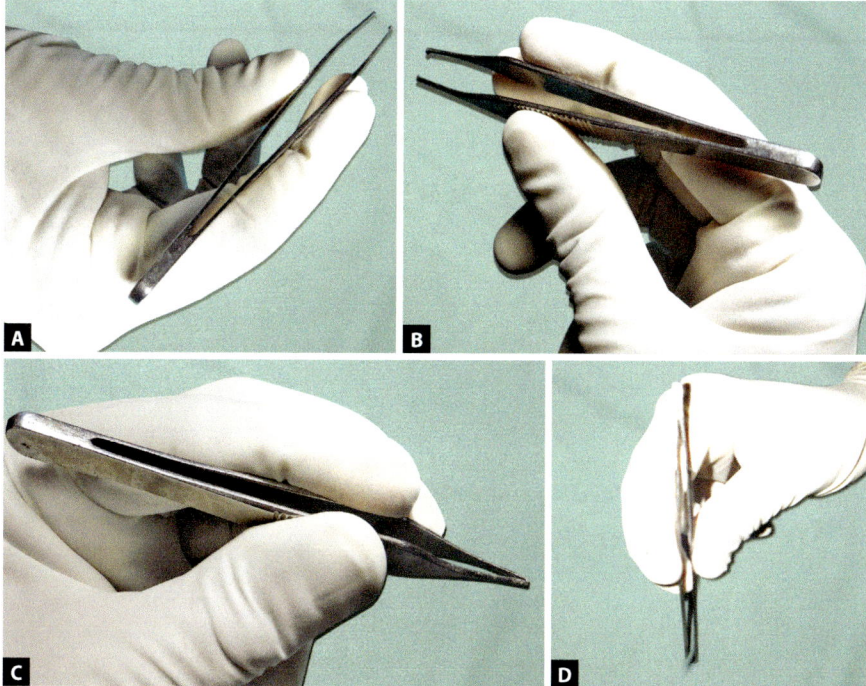

**Figs. 12A to D:** Technique of holding and using dissecting tissue forceps.

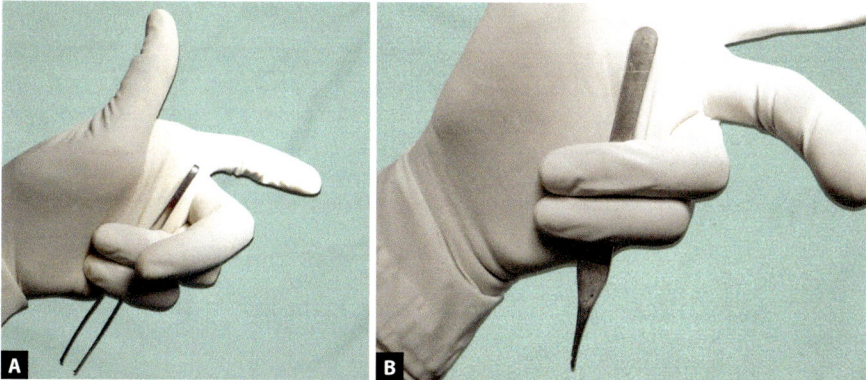

**Figs. 13A and B:** Forceps is placed in the palm (palming the forceps) while knotting the sutures after taking the bites.

or non-toothed. Skin and tough structures are held using toothed forceps. Muscle, fascia, bowel, and delicate structures are held using nontoothed forceps **(Figs. 12A to D)**. Tip may contain one or more apposing teeth in toothed forceps (one-in-two or two-in-three). Different vascular forceps are also available. Firm grip should be used to hold the tissue properly to prevent slippage and to allow passage of the needle across the tissue for suturing **(Figs. 13A and B)**.

### GAUZE

Gauze used can be woven or non-woven. In depth and wider fields mops are used.

*Non-woven gauze* can be made of natural materials such as cotton, linen, wood pulp, and paper or synthetic materials such as polyester, polypropylene, polyimide and polytetrafluoroethylene (PTFE). Non-wovens are usually lightweight, soft and flexible; offering precise absorbency, fluid retention porosity, low dust and shedding properties; allowing enhanced absorption and retention levels and also allow longer use. Cotton is natural, soft, comfortable, hypoallergenic and naturally absorbent with a greater wet than dry strength and is popular. Natural materials such as viscose, Tencel and lyocell (regenerated cellulose fibers often blended with polyamide or polyester materials) are also used. Biopolymer material like polylactide is new one with a renewable and biodegradable/recyclable option. Mops and gauzes are often having radiopaque lines as an identifying marker **(Fig. 14)**.

### SCALPEL HANDLE AND BLADE

*Bard Parker's handle* (BP handle) is a flat stainless steel (very sharp and resist dulling from frictions in tissues) or carbon steel (more sharp but prone for early dulling) instrument with a slot on narrower side on both surfaces to attach scalpel blade. 3, 4, 5, and 7 numbered blades are available. Number 4 handle is wider. Scalpel blades 10, 11, 12, and 15 fit in to Bard Parker handle numbers 3, 5, and 7. Scalpel blades 18, 19, 20, 21, 22, 23, and 24 fit into slot of Bard Parker's blade number 4. New blade is used into the slot of the handle for each

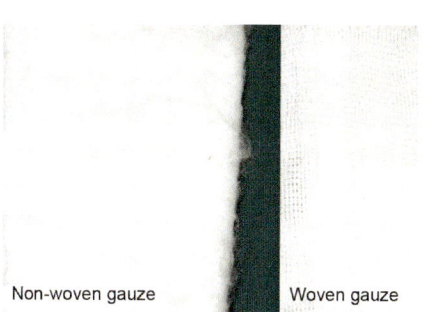

**Fig. 14:** Surgical gauze used during suturing.

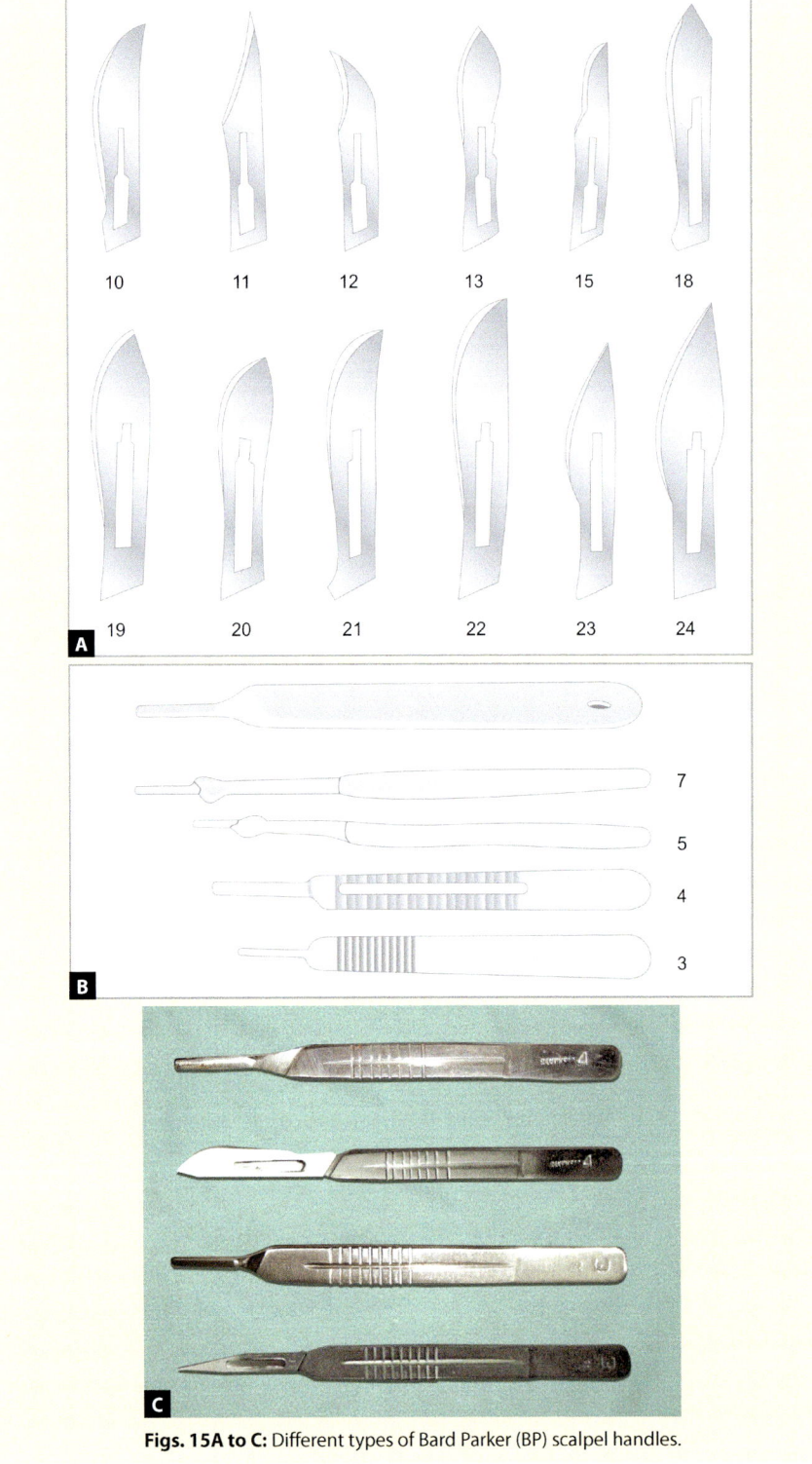

**Figs. 15A to C:** Different types of Bard Parker (BP) scalpel handles.

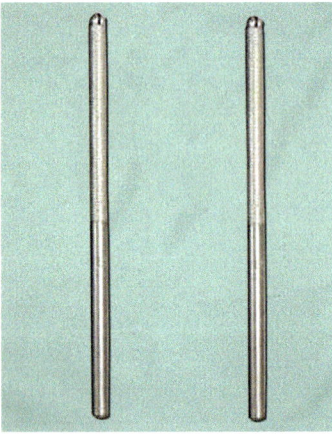

**Fig. 16:** Beaver handle is specialized knife handles which are used in fine incisions and in ophthalmology.

edge faces surgeon. Number 15 is used in plastic surgery, head and neck surgery, face surgeries. Numbers 20, 22, and 24 are used in skin incisions of major surgeries such as laparotomy, thoracotomy, craniotomy, and incisions in limb. Blades are sterilized by gamma radiation with aluminum foil packing. Commonly blades are used only once and then disposed. If sterilization is needed, then it is done by immersing in cetrimide/lysol solution (not autoclave or boiling). Scalpel is also used for dissections of fascial planes, raising skin flaps, hernial sac, etc. Fine lateral oblique strokes are used for such dissections. One should have a control over the depth of dissection. When scalpel is used in the abdomen like while cutting the bowel, it should be used in such a way that sharp edge of the blade should face forward so that to avoid inadvertent injury to deeper vital structures. Bowel is cut from mesenteric margin toward antimesenteric surface. Number 3 and 4 Bard Parker knives are used commonly for different detachable blades.

*Diamond knives* are used in ophthalmology—Handles are made from titanium and high-quality aluminum and blades are honed from gem-quality diamonds.

## SCISSORS

Scissors are used for tissue cutting, dissection, and cutting the suture removal. Curved scissor is used for dissection. Straight scissor of different types is used for suture cutting. Fine scissors with different curvatures are available and used depending on the need, field, and precision in surgery **(Figs. 17A and B)**.

## HEMOSTAT

Different types of hemostats are available—Medium-sized hemostat (artery forceps), large artery forceps, and Halsted fine

patient and so sharpness of the blade is maintained. BP handle is sterilized by autoclave. Disposable handles even though not commonly practiced are often used with attached blades. Number 3 BP handle with number 15 blade and number 4 handle with number 22, 21, or 10 blades. Number 7 BP handle works like number 3 allowing corresponding blades but is lengthier **(Figs. 15A to C)**. *Beaver handle* is another handle but needs specialized blades. It is used in microsurgery and in ophthalmology. 15C blade, a specialized one, is often used which is smaller than 15 blade **(Fig. 16)**.

Blades are usually of detachable one. Number 11 blade is a stab knife blade which is used in incision and drainage of an abscess and in making small incision like for drains. Number 12 blade is curved one, used for tonsillectomy. Here cutting

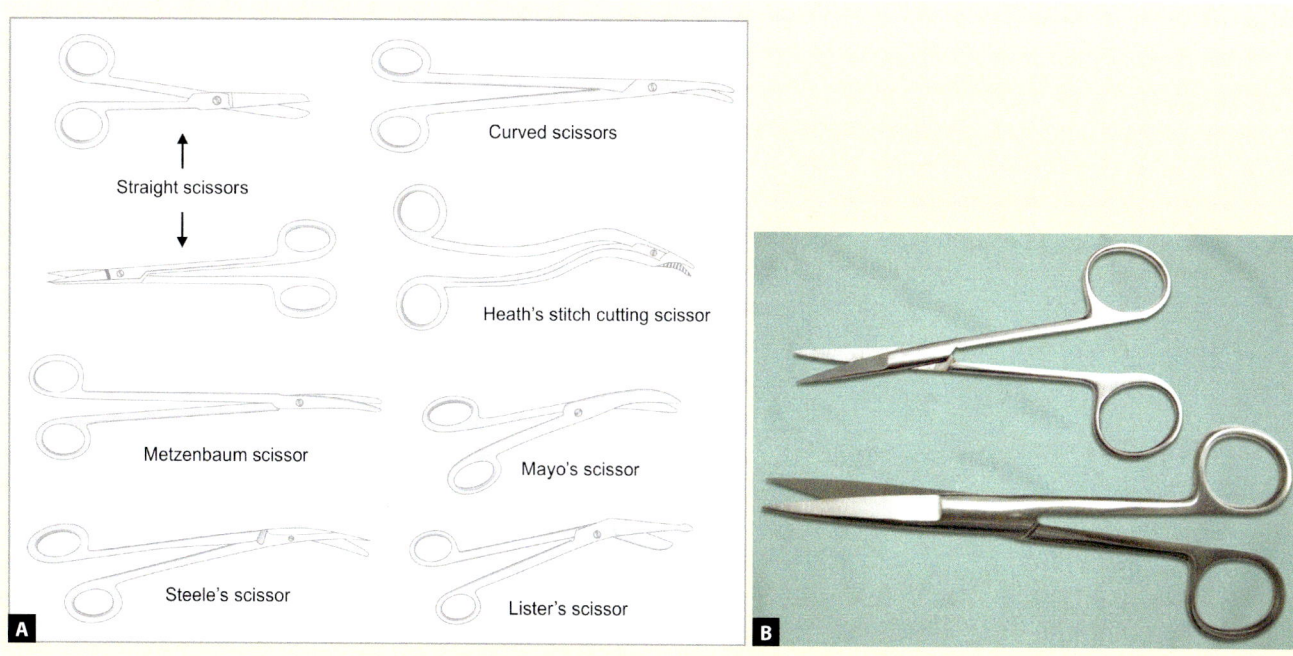

**Figs. 17A and B:** Different scissors used in surgical practice.

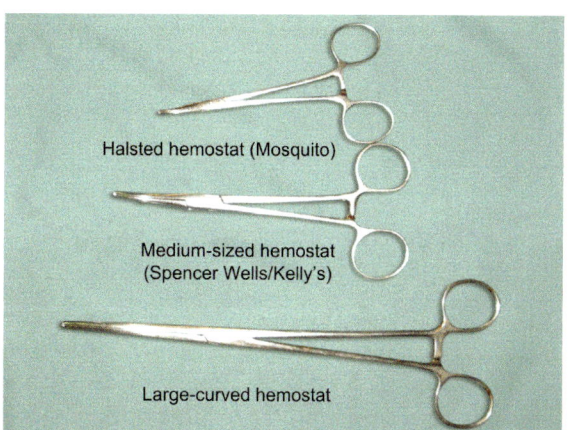

**Fig. 18:** Hemostats used during suturing to catch bleeders while suturing.

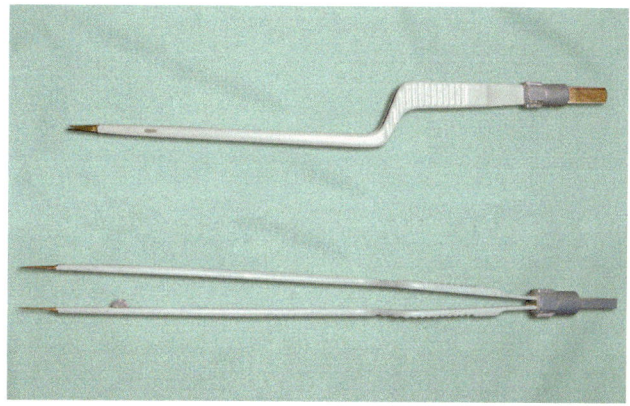

**Fig. 19:** Bayonet forceps with curves in the handle used in bipolar cautery. Bent and straight types are available.

mosquito forceps. It is used to catch the bleeders and to control hemorrhage **(Fig. 18)**.

## CAUTERY

Cautery is an essential tool in surgical field. Both monopolar and bipolar cautery are used. Bipolar is better for hemostasis which does not require earthling **(Figs. 19 and 20)**.

## SKIN STAPLER

It is a device to appose the skin wound edge by placing series of stapler pins. It is quick and saves time. It causes less inflammatory reaction and so less postoperative wound pain. Removal is easier using a specialized device. But it is not hemostatic; wound edge eversion cannot be achieved properly. It is used mainly after laparotomy, limb surgeries and in quick closure of lengthy skin wounds **(Figs. 21A to C)**. It is not much useful in cosmetic surgeries.

## SUTURE REMOVAL SET OR CLIP REMOVAL

Suture removal is done in skin sutures whether it is simple or mattress sutures. Absorbable suture (subcuticular) is usually not removed. Straight scissor is used for stitch removal. Heath's specialized scissor is also useful **(Figs. 22A to C)**. Toothed tissue forceps is essential to hold the knot ends (ears of the suture). Suture is cut away from the wound and pulled out toward the wound edge. 11 number blade also can be used to remove the stitch. Straight scissor is also used to cut the knot ends after knotting the suture. Curved scissor should be used to cut the tail ends of the knot in the depth and close to the vital structures. Suture area is first clean with normal saline. The suture is grasped with non-tooth dissecting forceps and lifted above the epithelial surface. Scissors are then passed through one loop and then transected close to the surface to avoid dragging contaminated suture materials through tissues. The suture is then pulled toward the incision line to prevent dehiscence **(Fig. 23)**. If suture entrapped in a scab, then application of hydrogen peroxide/normal saline is necessary. Clip removal is done with specific instrument which widens the clip ends outward and removes the clip-like a "W" **(Figs. 24 and 25)**.

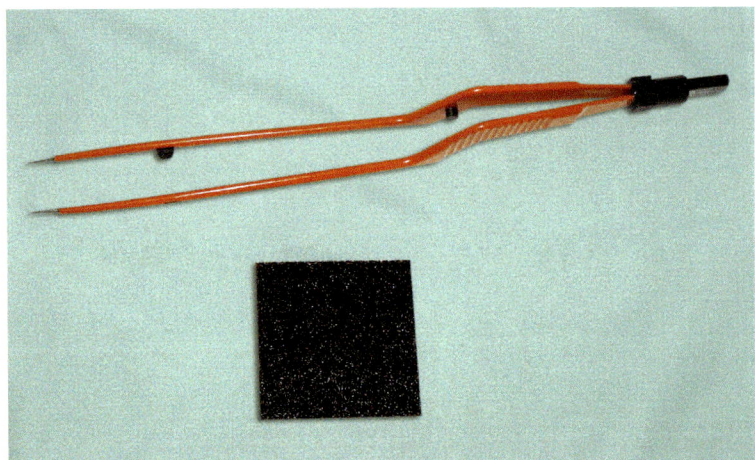

**Fig. 20:** Nonsticky bipolar cautery.

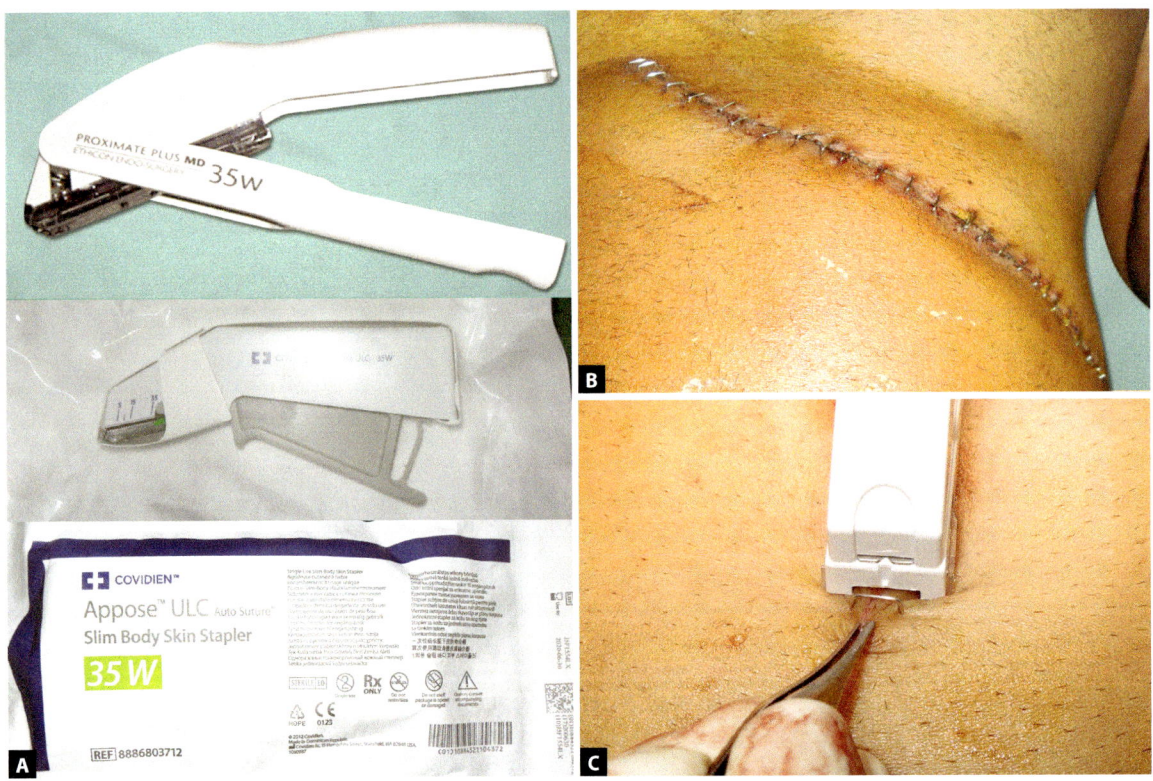

**Figs. 21A to C:** Skin stapler and stapled wound.

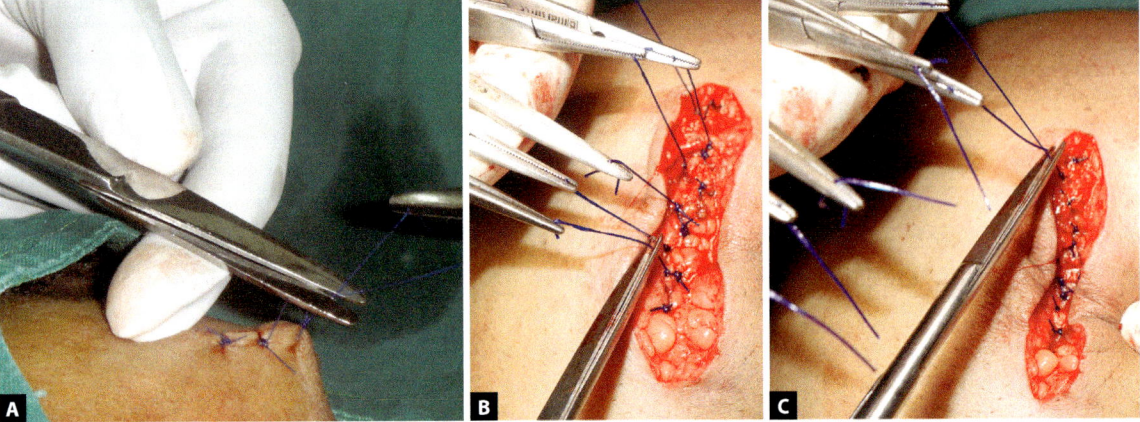

**Figs. 22A to C:** Straight scissor is used to cut the tails of the suture after knotting. 4-mm tail ends are left to avoid knot slippage and later to make suture removal easier.

## Instruments for Suturing

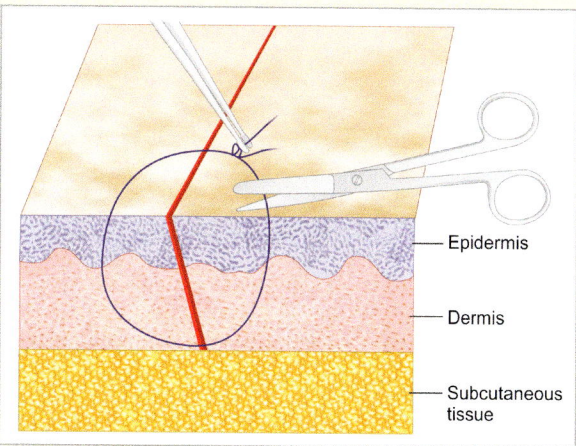

**Fig. 23:** Suture is removed after cutting the suture very close to skin surface on the opposite side of the wound; after cutting the knot that is held, it should be pulled toward the wound side, not away from the wound site. Both ends of the loop should not be cut; if done it will cause retaining of the suture material inside the wound creating complications.

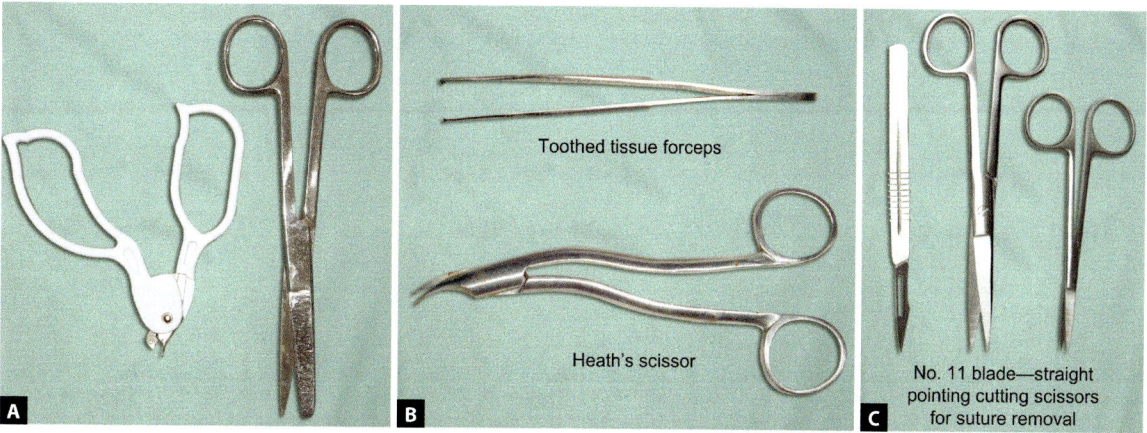

**Figs. 24A to C:** Clip removal and suture removal set.

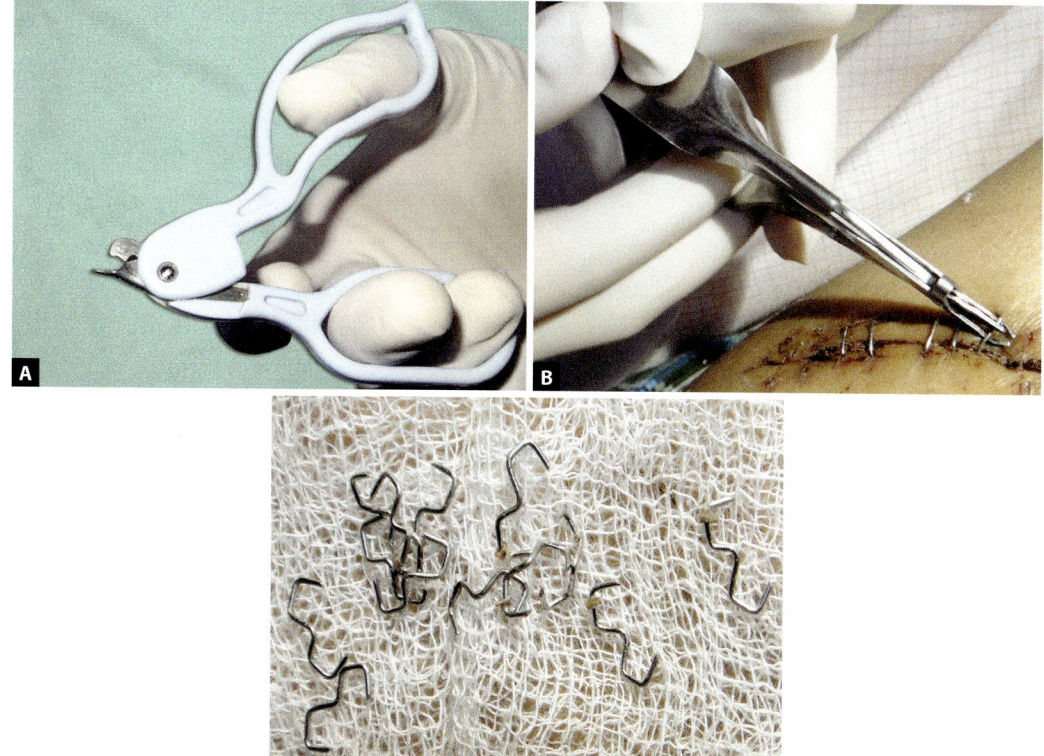

**Figs. 25A to C:** Skin stapler clip removal.

## LAPAROSCOPIC NEEDLE HOLDER (FIGS. 26A AND B)

Coaxial handle needle holder is better than pistol handle needle holder. Handle is ringless which facilitates better maneuverability. Handles are heavy and strong to have a firm grip. Tip is either straight or curved to place the needle. Only one of the jaws in the tip opens. Right and left hand needle holders (two-needle holders) are better to have easy suturing technique; but commonly we use needle holder in one hand and serrated non-toothed grasper or Maryland instrument in another. Tip with jaws should be strong and hold the needle firmly without any slippage during movements while taking bites from the tissues.

## BIOADHESIVES

Bioadhesive-like iso-amyl-2 cyanoacrylate is used for apposition of skin especially in small incisions, laparoscopic port-site incisions, etc. **(Fig. 27)**. Few adhesives materials are tried in fixing the synthetic material like mesh also.

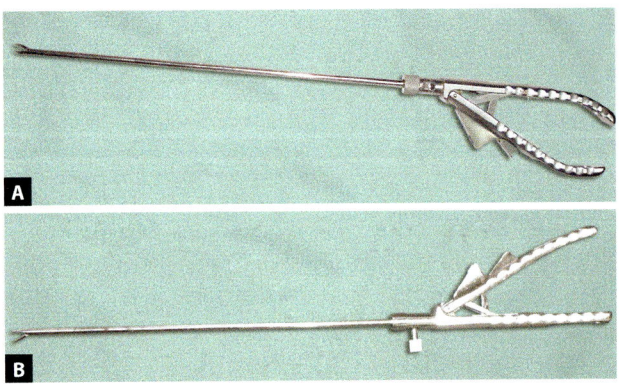

**Figs. 26A and B:** Laparoscopic needle holder.

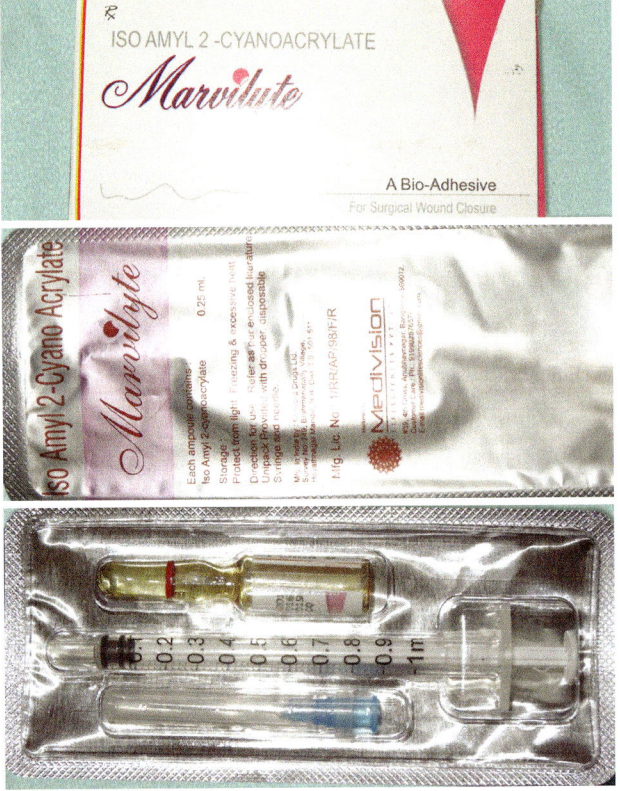

**Fig. 27:** Bioadhesive-like iso-amyl-2 cyanoacrylate is used for skin apposition in small incisions.

# CHAPTER 3: Suture Materials and Needles

> "We must turn to nature itself, to the observations of the body in health and disease, to learn the truth."
> —Hippocrates

## SUTURE MATERIALS

### INTRODUCTION

Definition and meanings of suture materials are described in different ways. Suture material is an artificial fiber/strand used to keep wound together until they hold sufficiently well by themselves by natural fiber (collagen) which is synthesized and woven into a stronger scar. Suture is a stitch/series of stiches made to secure apposition of the edges of a surgical wound—Wilkins. It is also defined as any strand of material utilized to ligate blood vessels or approximate tissues—Silverstein LH (1999).

Suture apposes the wound edges; support the tissues; reduces the pain; provides wound strength; can be hemostatic; and avoids exposure of deeper tissues such as bone, vessels, and nerves by covering them. It supports the tissues and gives sufficient strength to the wound until healing process is complete.

### CLASSIFICATION

Suture material is a foreign body used to appose and align the tissues and wounds either on the surface or in the deeper tissues. It tends to elicit some amount of foreign body reaction. Absolute aseptic precautions are required while suturing. Suture material is classified based on its origin, absorption, and structure.

*Natural suture materials* are derived from plant or animal sources. Natural suture materials cause more antigenicity and inflammatory reactions compared to synthetic one. Natural suture material gets absorbed by enzymatic degradation whereas synthetic one by hydrolysis. Natural sutures show good handling and knot-holding abilities but cause tissue reaction. No foreign body can be left permanently in the patient, which can cause possible long-term problems. *Synthetic sutures* are made by industrial process using polymers, polyamides, etc. They are less reactive and stronger. But handling is difficult with them and they may get expelled/extruded out by the body.

*Nonabsorbable sutures* offer longer duration of tensile strength than absorbable one. They give permanent wound support. *Absorbable one* gives temporary wound support until wound heals to withstand usual stress. Monofilament which is single-stranded filament shows least resistance during passage through tissues compared to multifilament suture which is multistranded. *Monofilament sutures* show least capillarity; are smooth and pass easily through tissues (less tissue drag) and carry less risk of tissue trauma and infection. But it has got high memory; handling and knotting is difficult with difficulty in knot burial. *Multifilament suture* offers higher tensile strength with better pliability, flexibility, handling and knot holding ability and secure knotting. But it has got increased capillarity and increased absorption of fluid and so infection can occur; it shows more tissue resistance (high tissue drag) and more tissue trauma.

### Absorbable

- *Natural—monofilament:* Catgut (natural amino acid polymer).
- *Synthetic:*
  - *Monofilament:* Poliglecaprone (monocryl); polyglyconate (Maxon); polydioxanone suture (PDS).
  - *Multifilament:* Coated polyglycolic acid (Dexon); Polyglactin-910; lactomer copolymer (polysorb).

### Nonabsorbable

- *Natural:*
  - *Monofilament*
  - *Multifilament:* Surgical silk (natural amino acid polymer), surgical linen (natural cellulose polymer), cotton, Ramie (Chinese fiber).
- *Metallic*—stainless steel—monofilament; stainless steel—multifilament.
- *Synthetic:*
  - *Monofilament:* Polypropylene, polyethylene, polyamide, polyester monofilament
  - *Multifilament:* Polyamide braided, polyester braided.

---

**Classification I**
- Coated
- Uncoated

**Classification II**
- *Monofilament:* Catgut, poliglecaprone, polyglyconate, PDS, polypropylene, polyethylene
- *Multifilament:*
  - *Braided:* Silk, polyamide braided, Polyglactin-910, Dexon
  - *Twisted:* Cotton, linen

---

*Monofilament suture materials* (single-stranded) are smooth, strong and least reactive which will not allow bacteria to harbor. But handling and knot holding properties are poor **(Fig. 1)**. Polypropylene shows good memory. Recoiling tendency of the suture material is called as *'memory'* of the suture material. Higher the memory difficult in handling and knotting. Lesser the memory means better the handling quality.

*Multifilament sutures* (multistranded with multiple filaments) are easier to handle with less memory **(Fig. 1 and Table 1)**. But they may harbor bacteria easily and are not suitable in infected field. They cause more reaction to tissues.

---

*Features of ideal suture material **(Figs. 2A to G)***
- It should be least reactive, should not allow harboring of the bacteria.
- It should be nonelectrolytic, noncapillary, nonallergenic, and noncarcinogenic.
- It should have good/high tensile strength (uniform tensile strength).
- It should have uniform diameter and size.
- It should have pliability for proper knot holding with easy handling ability.
- It should achieve good knot security.
- It should have low capillarity; multifilament sutures have high capillarity causing more infection.
- It should have favorable absorption in relation to the tissue where it is needed.
- It should have good BSR (breaking strength retention).
- It can be used in any tissue—tissue biocompatibilty.
- It should have low modulus of elasticity.
- It should have less memory. *Memory* is inherent capacity of the suture material to return to or maintain its original gross shape which is related to plasticity, pliability, and diameter.
- It should be amenable for proper sterilization without deterioration of its properties.
- It should be easily available and cheaper.

*Note:* No suture material will be having 100% ideal features; polypropylene and polyglactin-910 are excellent suture materials used widely worldwide.

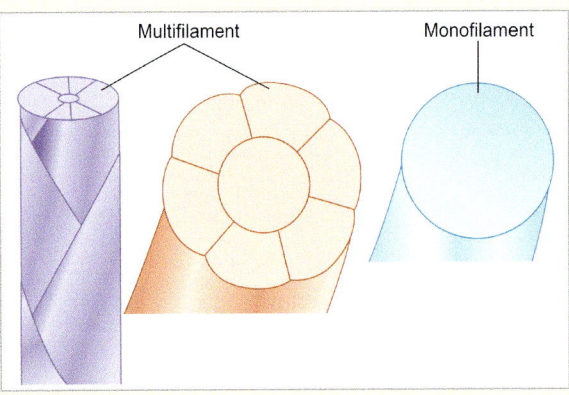

**Fig. 1:** Suture materials—multifilament and monofilament.

**Table 1:** Characteristics of suture materials—multifilament and monofilament.

| Monofilament | Multifilament |
|---|---|
| • Handling is difficult | • Handling is easier |
| • Knot holding is difficult | • Knotting is easier |
| • Smooth and strong | • Less strength |
| • No wicking | • Wicking is problem |
| • Thinner | • Thicker |
| • No bacterial harbor | • Bacteria can harbor |
| • No capillarity | • Capillarity is common |
| • Stretching and crimping is the problem | |

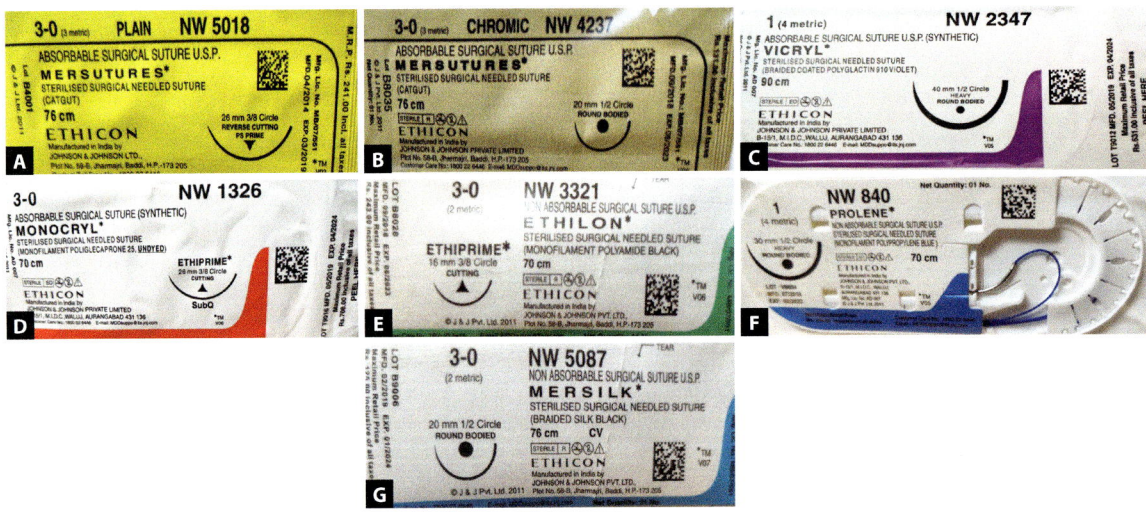

**Figs. 2A to G:** Different suture materials used in surgical practice.

## PROPERTIES OF THE SUTURE MATERIAL (FIG. 3)

- *Mechanical properties* are assessed using tensiometer (Instrom machine) by recording stress strain curve evaluating the yield stress, breaking stress and modulus of the elasticity.
- *Biological properties* are biodegradability, tissue reaction, tissue incorporation, infection rate, material deposition such as calcium on to the placed suture material. It depends on the chemical nature of the suture material, type of material (mono- or multifilament), surface charge on the suture material.
- *Surgical properties* are handling, tissue sliding, tensile strength, knot run down and knot holding (knot security).

*Note:* Details about the suture material are printed in the wrap; one should carefully read it before use.

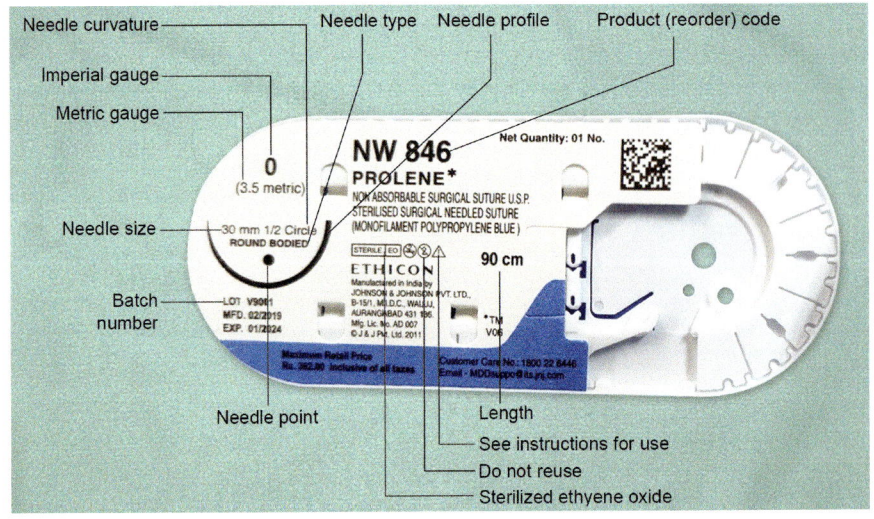

**Fig. 3:** One should know how to read instructions of the package wrap.

## BIOLOGY OF SUTURE MATERIALS

As suture material is a foreign body, both cellular response and enzymatic activity occur together. Tissue reaction is more to natural absorbable suture material than synthetic absorbable suture material. Plain catgut shows more tissue reaction than chromic catgut. Tissue reaction is more toward silk, linen or cotton compared to polyamide, polyester or polypropylene (least).

The initial body response to sutures is almost identical in the first 4–7 days, regardless of the suture material. The early response is a generalized acute aseptic inflammation, involving primarily polymorphonuclear leukocytes. After few days mononuclear cells, fibroblasts and histiocytes will be prominent. Capillary formation occurs later. Natural absorbable suture undergoes proteolytic degradation with intense tissue response; synthetic absorbable undergoes hydrolysis and is less intense; and nonabsorbable suture undergoes encapsulation with acellular response.

Sutures passing through mucous membrane or skin provide a "wick" or pathway through which bacteria track down, and bacteria gain access to underlying tissues. The longer the suture remains, the deeper the epithelial invasion of the underlying tissue. When suture removed, epithelial tract remains and these cells may eventually disappear or remain to form keratin and epithelial inclusion cysts. The epithelial pathway results in typical *"railroad scar"* formation.

## Suture Tensile Strength

It is breaking strength of the suture material, which is important in holding tissues in approximated position during stages of wound healing. Inadequate tensile strength or rapid loss of tensile strength may result in disruption of the suture line. As apposed tissue needs at least initial 7 days to regain its tensile strength, at least for 7 days tissues should be kept in apposition by suture material. It is actually a measure of tissue's ability to resist deformation and breakage.

*Tensile strength* is the one which holds the tissues in approximation until tissue wound heals strongly. So adequate tensile strength is an essential component of a suture material. *Breaking strength* of a suture material is expressed either in grams per denier (weight of a fiber per 9,000 m length) or newtons per tex (weight of a fiber per 1,000 m length). It is also related to the size and diameter of the suture material **(Table 2)**. *Wound breaking strength* is limit of tensile strength of a healing wound at which separation of the wound edges occur.

## Breaking Strength Retention

Breaking strength retention is related to the rate and extent of the biodegradability of the suture. It is studied by immersing the suture in fluids as in vitro BSR or putting into animal tissues as in vivo BSR. It reflects the duration of the tensile strength maintained in the tissue beyond which suture fails.

## Elasticity of the Suture Material

It is the ability to deform or stretch when suture is subjected to a progressive distraction force and inability to reach back to its original dimension even after force is removed beyond yield point. It is the measure of the ability of the suture material to regain its original form and length after deformation.

## Capillarity

It is the extent to which absorbed fluid is transferred along the suture material. *Fluid absorption:* It is the ability of the suture material to take up fluid after immersion.

## Knot-pull Tensile Strength

It is the breaking strength of knotted suture material (10–40% weaker after deformation by knot placement); *Knot strength:* It is the amount of force necessary to cause a knot to slip. *Straight pull tensile strength:* It is the linear breaking strength of the suture material.

## Plasticity

It is the measure of the ability to deform without breaking and to maintain a new form after relief of the deforming force. *Pliability:* It is the ease of handling of suture material so that knot tension can be adjusted and secure knots can be placed comfortably.

## Absorption Time

It is not equal to tensile strength period. It is progressive loss of volume of the suture material. Absorption of suture material may be rapid or delayed or slow. Ideally tensile strength and absorption time should last for at least 3 weeks to have an efficient tissue apposition. Catgut gets absorbed by cellular response and phagocytosis; synthetic absorbable suture gets absorbed by hydrolysis using tissue fluids.

*Absorption of suture materials:* Suture material is degraded either by enzymatic process as in gut sutures, or by hydrolysis as in many of the synthetic materials such as glycolic acid, ployglactin-910 or polydioxanone. Nonabsorbable sutures are walled off or encapsulated. In infected tissues or in a patient with protein

**Table 2:** Size and diameter of the suture material.

| Size in mm—gauge | Suture diameter in mm | Metric size—Metric number is diameter of the suture in 10ths of an mm | Needle diameter | Suture diameter | Needle to suture ratio |
|---|---|---|---|---|---|
| 2 | 0.57 | 5.0 | 1,400 µm | 570 µm | 2.4:1 |
| 1 | 0.47 | 4.0 | 1,100 µm | 470 µm | 2.3:1 |
| 0 | 0.40 | 3.5 | 900 µm | 400 µm | 2.2:1 |
| 2/0 | 0.34 | 3.0 | 750 µm | 340 µm | 2.2:1 |
| 3/0 | 0.25 | 2.0 | 650 µm | 250 µm | 2.6:1 |
| 4/0 | 0.20 | 1.5 | 500 µm | 200 µm | 2.5:1 |
| 5/0 | 0.15 | 1.0 | 400 µm | 150 µm | 2.7:1 |
| 6/0 | 0.11 | 0.7 | 300 µm | 110 µm | 2.7:1 |
| 7/0 | 0.07 | 0.5 | 250 µm | 070 µm | 3.6:1 |
| 8/0 | 0.05 | 0.4 | 200 µm | 45 µm | 4.44:1 |
| 9/0 | 0.035 | 0.3 | 140 µm | 35 µm | 4.0:1 |
| 10/0 | 0.022 | 0.2 | 70 µm | 22 µm | 3.18:1 |

deficiency, suture breakdown may be accelerated. If the loss of tensile strength outpaces the healing phase, failure of the wound results. It causes wound disruption. Absorbable suture materials get absorbed from 7 to 60 days. Nonabsorbable suture material loses its tensile strength only from 60 days to 2 years. Polypropylene maintains its strength as late as 2 years.

*Note:* Size zero or/and 1-0 are same.

## ABSORBABLE SUTURES

### Natural Absorbable Suture

Plain and chromic catgut, collagen sutures, Cargile membrane, fascia lata, and Kangaroo tendon are different natural absorbable sutures. Only catgut is used now. Collagen suture is derived from Tendo Achilles of cattle containing 100% collagen; its action is similar such as catgut but it is stiffer; it is no longer used. Cargile membrane is derived from submucosa of cecum or peritoneum of ox. It was once practiced to cover removed pleura or peritoneum or to prevent adhesions after abdominal surgery. It is also no longer used. Fascia lata is derived from same individual's thigh or from cattle. It was once used in hernia repair, in correction of drooping of the upper eyelid and in facial palsy. Kangaroo tendon is derived from the tendons of the tail of the kangaroos. It shows high tensile strength but is no more in use.

### Catgut

It is monofilament natural absorbable suture material. It is derived from submucosa of jejunum of sheep or serosa of cattle intestine. It contains *99% collagen—protein* by nature. It gets absorbed by enzymatic degradation by proteolytic enzymes derived from macrophages. In the presence of infection catgut is rapidly absorbed. It can be plain or chromic catgut (treated with chromic acid). Heat treated fast absorbing gut is also available. Fast absorbing gut is used often in transepidermal suturing wherein suture removal is not necessary and impractical. Fast absorbing gut should only be used for skin not in deeper tissues. Plain catgut causes more reaction but for shorter period compared to chromic catgut. Plain catgut loses its tensile strength completely in 7-15 days; chromic catgut in 30 days. Tissue reaction is early and rapid in plain and slower in chromic catgut. Handling and knot holding property is good in catgut. Plain catgut is straw-colored and chromic is brown-colored. Plain catgut is wet whereas chromic catgut gets dried fast (so it is smooth). Plain catgut is used in apposition of the subcutaneous tissue, ligating bleeders in the subcutaneous tissue and often in circumcision. Chromic catgut is used in obstetric and gynecological surgeries such as cesarean or ligation of pedicles in hysterectomy. Catgut is ideal for *surgical slip knots* due to its rough texture which imparts an intrinsic resistance for reverse slipping. So, it is commonly used as endo-loops in laparoscopic surgeries such as in laparoscopic appendicectomy. Sterile dry packed chromic catgut is suitable for slip knot. Alcohol-packed chromic catgut once unpacked can be made dry if left for 15 minutes. It is used also in suturing the muscle, ligating pedicles in infected field, etc. Earlier atraumatic straight needled chromic catgut was popular in bowel anastomosis but is no longer advocated. Many of catgut uses are replaced by other synthetic absorbable sutures.

It is manufactured as follows—after washing, intestine is slit longitudinally into four strands; muscle and fat are removed using water spray—*sliming*. Chemical bath saponification is also used to remove fat. Strands are spun together, dried with tension and electronically polished. It is absorbed by inflammatory reaction and phagocytosis.

It is the oldest known absorbable suture; Galen referred to gut suture as early as 175 AD. It is derived from sheep intestinal submucosa or bovine intestinal serosa. Submucosa of sheep has a rich elastic tissue content which accounts for high tensile strength of the catgut. It is monofilament and is available in the plain form as well as "tanned" in chromic acid. The tanning process delays the digestion by white blood cell lysozymes.

*Chromic catgut* is catgut with chromic acid salt. The catgut is treated with 20% chromium salt in water with five parts of glycerine. It is brown in color. Its absorption time is 21 days. It is used in suturing muscle, fascia, external oblique aponeurosis, ligating pedicles, etc. Atraumatic sutures are manufactured either by swaging or by entangling the suture material in to the grooved proximal part of the needle by mechanical pressure. Winded suture material in a support card is packed in a foil envelope with isopropyl alcohol. It is sterilized by gamma radiation.

Catgut should not be boiled or autoclaved as heat destroys its tensile strength. Catgut is sterilized during preparation and kept in a preservative solution (isopropyl alcohol) inside spools or foils. Unused and reusable catgut is hygroscopic so, catgut will swell due to water absorption and its tensile strength will be reduced.

### Synthetic Absorbable Sutures

They are polymers and carbohydrate by nature, absorbed by hydrolysis. They can be monofilament or multifilament—braided. Braiding may be either looping or in multiplicity. They maintain higher tensile strength and so keep the approximation stronger for longer period. They are usually pliable, smooth, glides along the tissues smoothly.

They are biodegradable by hydrolysis and less reactive with easy handling property with less memory. They can be monofilament or multifilament suture materials. PDS, polyglyconate (Maxon), poliglecaprone (Monocryl), biosyn, and Caprosyn are monofilament types of synthetic absorbable sutures. Coated polyglycolic acid (Dexon), polyglactin (polyglycolide co-lactide; polyglactin-910), and lactomer copolymer (polysorb) are multifilament absorbable suture materials.

### *Polyglyconate (Maxon, Davis and Geck)*

It is *monofilament absorbable* synthetic suture material which is absorbed by hydrolysis releasing glycolic acid and hydrogen ion which lowers the pH in the tissue and so least infection rate. *It is a copolymer of glycolic acid and trimethylene carbonate.* It lasts longer period taking around 6 months to get absorbed. It shows good handling features in both open surgery and laparoscopy. Its dyed color is visible and stains under the skin. It shows excellent tensile strength, knot holding property and minimum memory. Its tensile strength is more than dexon. It gets absorbed by hydrolysis in 180 days. In vitro studies by Edlich and co-workers (1973) have suggested that the degradation products of polyglycolic acid and nylon sutures—glycolic acid, 1,6-hexane diamine and adipic acid are antibacterial agents.

### *Glycomer-631 (Biosyn, Covidien)*

It is *monofilament absorbable* synthetic suture material showing good handling features and tensile strength. Its absorption is slow; taking 4 months to get absorbed.

### *Polyglytone-621 (Caprosyn)*

It is *fast absorbing monofilament* synthetic suture material which is absorbed in 8 weeks and its tensile strength lasts for 10 days only. So it is used in suturing low tension approximations. It contains glycolide, caprolactone, trimethylene carbonate and lactide. It achieves secure wound approximation with excellent handling and knot holding property with least reaction. It is used for soft tissue approximation but not in cardiovascular/neurological/ophthalmologic surgeries.

### *Poliglecaprone-25 (Monocryl, Ethicon)*

It is *monofilament absorbable* synthetic suture material with excellent handling features with smooth surface, pliable (less stiff and less hard), adequate knot holding property causing minimal tissue reaction. This suture material is very easy to bend and to stretch. Gliding and passage through tissues is smooth and less dragging and so minimizes the trauma to tissues. It is copolymer of 75% glycolide and 25% caprolactone. It shows high tensile strength for 3 weeks and absorbed by hydrolysis in 90 days. It does not have package memory and so recoiling and inadvertent knotting is not present. Proper tissue sliding, adequate elasticity, ideal handling, and visible transparent color make it as ideal absorbable monofilament suture material. It is sterilized by ethylene oxide. It is the most pliable suture material ever made.

### Polydioxanone Suture Material

It is the *strongest monofilament absorbable* suture material which lasts longer period maintaining its tensile strength in the wound. It is nonreactive, absorbable, synthetic suture material. It contains polymerized paradioxanone 97%; 3% copolymerized lactide. It is absorbed by hydrolysis (in 6 months). PDS-II is improvized version of the PDS-I in relation to handling property. PDS glides through tissues well but can cause crinkling. It is very good for open surgery but not suitable for endoscopic surgery. Absorption begins in 90 days and completes in 6 months. *V Loc* is the barbed suture which is self-anchoring and no knots are required; it contains 0 number PDS material with axially barbed segments. It passes through tissues easily; shows minimum tissue reaction; knot holding and security is good; useful in wounds under tension and contaminated wounds; gives very effective wound support for >60 days. But it may get extruded through wounds due to delay in absorption.

### Polyglactin-910 (Vicryl, Ethicon)

It is *braided, multifilament*, synthetic, coated *absorbable* suture material which is a polymer made up of glycolic acid with lactide component. Ratio is 9 of polyglycolic acid to 1 lactide. Lactide being hydrophobic reduces the water molecule ingress into the copolymer preventing the breakdown of the linkage of the glycolic acid copolymer chain thereby increasing the longevity of the suture material and its tensile strength. Lactide reduces the regularity and crystallinity of the copolymer making it to have greater pliability. Water repelling property of lactide slows down the loss of tensile strength. Polyglactin shows more tensile strength and handling character than many other suture materials. Coated polyglactin suture material contains 50% polyglactin (Polyglactin coat component contains 35% polyglycolide and 65% lactide) and 50% calcium stearate (it is an absorbable fatty acid lubricant). This coating reduces the surface friction of the braided suture material without altering the quality of the suture material like absorption, reaction, and tensile strength. It is absorbed by hydrolysis (not protein degradation) and so least reactive. It gets absorbed in 90 days and maintains tensile strength for 30 days. It shows superior pliability, less tissue drag with adequate wound support. It is sterilized by ethylene oxide. It is stored in an optimum temperature below 25°C. Life of packed material is 5 years.

Polyglactin-910 (Vicryl) is the most commonly used suture material in all open surgeries and in laparoscopic surgeries. It is not used in cardiovascular and neural suturing. Rapidly absorbing type (Vicryl rapid; velosorb fast) is also available which gets absorbed in 2 weeks. Antibacterial polyglactin (Vicryl plus) suture material is also often used. *Triclosan* is nontoxic, noncarcinogenic, antibacterial agent (not antibiotic) which is safe and effective and is used to protect the suture material from bacterial colonization (Vicryl plus). *Triclosan* on Vicryl plus creates a zone of inhibition around the suture.

### Coated Polyglycolic Acid (Dexon II, Davis and Geck)

It is polyglycolic acid with bioabsorbable copolymer of polyoxypropylene and polyoxyethylene coated with polycaprolate multifilament braided suture material. Its features are almost similar to polyglactin.

### Lactomer Copolymer—Polysorb

It is *braided, multifilament*, and synthetic *absorbable* suture material which consists of glycolide and lactide (93.5 : 6.5). It is coated with glycolide and caprolactone. It is suitable for both open and laparoscopic and for both interrupted and continuous suturing. It has got good tensile strength, tissue glide, knot holding capacity, easy handling properties. It gets absorbed in 3 months. But being purple in color it shows poor visibility. It is very useful for laparoscopic suturing and extracorporeal slip knot placement. Glycolide provides initial tensile strength but gets hydrolyzed rapidly; lactide provides prolonged tensile strength with slow hydrolysis.

> *Uses of absorbable suture materials:*
> - In bowel anastomosis such as gastro-jejunostomy, resection, and anastomosis—Vicryl (2-0) is used.
> - In cholecysto-jejunostomy (CCJ), choledocho-jejunostomy (CDJ)—Vicryl is used.
> - In suturing muscle, fascia, peritoneum, subcutaneous tissue, mucosa.
> - In ligating pedicles, e.g., ligation of pedicles during hysterectomy. 1-0 chromic catgut or Vicryl are used.
> - In circumcision usually 3-0 plain or chromic catgut or Vicryl rapid are used.
> 
> Absorbable suture materials should not be used in suturing tendon, nerves, vessels (vascular anastomosis) or in hernia surgery where tissue approximation under stress is needed.

## NONABSORBABLE SUTURE MATERIALS

### Natural

#### Silk

Silk is *natural, nonabsorbable, multifilament, braided* suture material. Silk is derived from cocoon of the silkworm larvae (**Figs. 4A and B**). Silk is protein by nature. It is coated with a wax which reduces the capillary action. It causes cellular tissue reaction; it shows very high tensile strength which is lost in 2 years. It has got very good handling and knot holding property. It is sterilized by gamma irradiation. It is available as atraumatic eyeless needled sutures, precut (sutupak) sutures, with micropoint needles for ophthalmologic surgeries. Each filament is processed to remove the natural waxes and sericin gum. After braiding, the strands are dyed, stretched and impregnated with

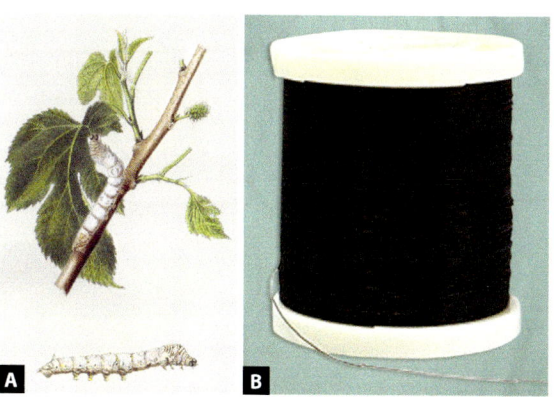

**Figs. 4A and B:** Silkworm—silk suture material is derived from it. (A) Silkworm; (B) Silk-braided roll.

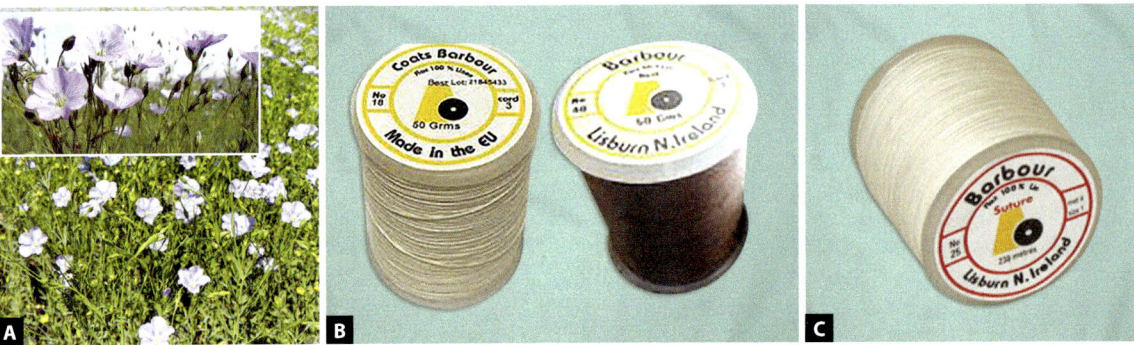

**Figs. 5A to C:** (A) Flax tree is used to get linen; (B and C) Barbour suture material (derived from linen/flax). It is strong, durable, can be sterilized by boiling, can be used in many areas such as suturing through eyed needle, ligatures, and anastomoses.

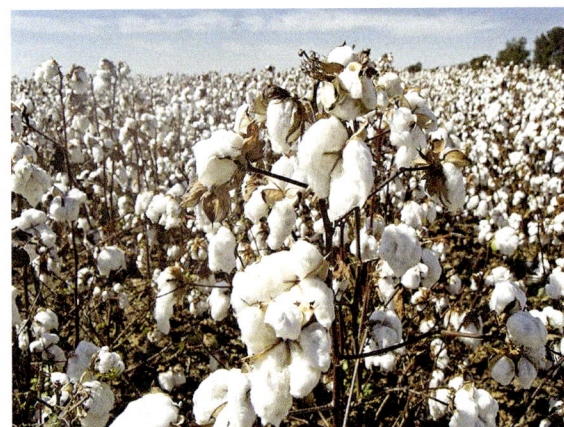

**Fig. 6:** Egyptian cotton tree.

a mixture of waxes and silicone. Dry silk suture is stronger than wet silk suture.

*Advantage:* Ease of handling as it is braided; good knot security; made noncapillary in order to withstand action of body fluids and moisture (due to wax and silicon coat); it is cost effective.

*Contraindications:* It should not be used in presence of infection.

*Linen*

It is *natural, nonabsorbable, multifilament, and twisted* suture material. Linen is a cellulose material derived from the flax (linseed) **(Fig. 5A)**. *Flax* is blue-flowered plant that is grown for its seed and textile fibers; textile fiber is made from the stalk of this tree used as a twisted multifilament suture material. It has got very good handling and knot holding property. Its tensile strength increases by 100% when it is wet. It is commonly used for ligatures, to tie pedicles. Barbour-linen thread is used in surgical suturing/ligatures. It is very strong with good knot holding property **(Figs. 5B and C)**. It is available as 20, 30, 35, 40, 60, 80, and 100 measurements. Here increase in number finer and thinner the suture material.

*Cotton*

It is *natural, nonabsorbable, and multifilament twisted* suture material derived from the hairs of the seed of the stable Egyptian cotton plant **(Fig. 6)**. It shows good knot security but not good in presence of contaminated wounds or infection. It is mainly used in ligating tissues and vessels.

### Synthetic

Synthetic nonabsorbable suture materials are hydrocarbon polymers derived from oil and coal. They are biocompatible usually non-biodegradable or slowly biodegradable and do not swell in the tissues. They show high flexibility and tensile strength, inertness, resistance to creep, and low melting point. But they have got poor knot retaining ability and knot may spill after placing. Usually they are monofilament but multifilament materials are available like polyester; multifilament is created by braiding from a multiplicity of monofilaments or by looping of a single filament.

*Nylon (New York, London)*

It is *polyamide* usually monofilament, synthetic, nonabsorbable suture material. It has got good tensile strength with minimal tissue reaction. But it shows high memory and so recoiling tendency and knot holding difficulty is common and so needs 4–5 throws to place the knot. It is slowly biodegradable. Polyamide suture (Ethilon, Ethicon; Dermalon, Davis and Geck) is available as atraumatic sutures and as sutupak sutures. Polyamide multifilament sutures are also available. Braided, sealed with silicone coating is also available but not found to be better than its monofilament counterpart.

*Dacron and Terylene/Polyesters*

They are *polyester* synthetic, nonabsorbable, multifilament, and braided sutures with high tensile strength with least reaction. But it has got a tendency to cut through; so Teflon® or polytetrafluoroethylene (PTFE) coating is provided.

*Ethibond* is polyester suture coated with polybutylate which prevents increase in diameter of the suture material and avoids flake in the tissues. Ethibond has got eight carrier molecules. Newer version, *ethibond excel* has got 16 carrier molecules which is smoother and better. It is used in cardiovascular and neurological surgeries. It is available in white and green colors to facilitate suturing in valve surgeries. It is very useful for slip knots in extracorporeal slip knot in laparoscopic surgeries.

*Polypropylene*

It is *monofilament, nonabsorbable, and synthetic suture material*. It has got high tensile strength with least reaction. It slides down through tissues easily but has got high memory with recoiling tendency and needs minimum five throws to have a secure knot. It is less thrombogenic and inert. It does not adhere to tissues. It is elastic and can fracture by undue grasping with forceps. It has got high fragility and plasticity. It shows high degree of smoothness with reasonable elasticity. It is highly visible in the wound. It has got uniform diameter. It is commonly used in all repairs such as hernia, vascular and neural anastomosis, and tendon suturing. It is used in pancreaticojejunostomy, often in pedicle ligations. It is used to close abdominal wall and repairs. It will not get weakened so easily; its tensile strength remains for 2 years. It is useful in infected field also. Suture pulling though the tissues is easier and quicker. It is least degradable. Surgipro-II is polypropylene with increased resistance for fraying so that better knot run down is achieved.

### Polyethylene

It is not commonly used as it is not as strong as other synthetic suture materials. It is a polymer by nature. It stretches and has got poor knot holding property.

### Expanded Polytetrafluoroethylene (Gore-Tex®)

It is a nonabsorbable, synthetic, monofilament suture material from expanded polytetrafluoroethylene (ePTFE) with least reaction, better handling, with good knot tensile strength and porous microstructure. It is used in all types of soft tissue approximation and cardiovascular surgeries. It is good suture material but is not commonly used.

### Polybutester–Novafil

It is monofilament, blue-colored, and synthetic suture material which has got adequate flexibility, suppleness and strength. Polybutester suture is a monofilament containing copolymer containing butylene terephthalate and polytetramethylene ether glycol (polyglycol trephthate and polybutylene terephthalate and is considered as a modified polyester suture). It, with low forces, yields greater elongation and the elasticity is superior allowing the suture to return to its original length once the load is removed. This unique feature of its ability to elongate or stretch with increasing wound edema and when edema subsides, suture resumes original shape makes it an ideal suture for lacerations with blunt trauma. It has no significant memory compared to polypropylene and nylon. It is easier to manipulate and greater knot security. Its high tensile strength with longevity and least tissue reaction makes it more and more popular.

### Polyvinylidene Fluoride

Polyvinylidene fluoride (PVDF) represents an attractive alternative to polypropylene as a monofilament vascular suture because of its satisfactory physicochemical properties, its ease of handling, and its good biocompatibility. It is monofilament, inert, ease handing property with knot security and compatible.

### Stainless Steel Metallic Nontoxic Suture/Wire (Steel, Tantalum, and Silver)

They are useful in approximating bones and tough structures, in neurosurgery, orthopedic, and thoracic surgeries (sternotomy or thoracotomy), in reconstructive surgeries, surgeries of skull base or head and neck, sinus surgeries, in dental surgeries. It is an alloy of iron, chromium, and nickel molybdenum. Monofilament is called as steel suture/metallic suture. Multifilament is called as metallic/steel wire which can be twisted or braided (**Fig. 7**). Metallic sutures/wires are difficult to handle and to use, may cause injury to surgeons but they have very high tensile strength and low reactivity. Kinking, electrolytic problems are—other problems. 18-gauge (*Brown and sharpe-gauge system*) is the largest; 40-gauge is the smallest diameter. It has got good tensile strength even in infection. But it is difficult to handle and has tendency to cut through tissues; very hard to tie, and knot ends require special handling. It has potential to corrode or break at points of twisting, bending or knotting. It cannot be used with prosthesis of another alloy. It is used in abdominal wall and skin closure, sternal closure, retention, tendon repair, orthopedic and neurosurgery; OMFS—for suspension of splints or arch bars.

*Disadvantages:* Linear artifacts caused by substances with high atomic number on CT images; possible movement of metal suture during MRI; and nickel sensitivity (patch test should be done).

> *According to USP (27th edition) nonabsorbable suture is classified and typed as follows (**Fig. 8**):*
>
> *Class-I:* It is composed of silk or synthetic fibers of monofilament, twisted or braided construction where the coating if any, does not significantly affect thickness (e.g., braided silk, polyester or nylon; monofilament nylon or polypropylene).
>
> *Class-II:* It is composed of cotton or linen fibers or coated natural or synthetic fibers where the coating significantly affects thickness but does not contribute significantly to strength (e.g., virgin-silk suture).
>
> *Class-III:* It is suture composed of monofilament or multifilament metal wire.

### Barbed Suture

It is knotless surgical suture which has barbs on its surface which once penetrates the tissue locks the suture preventing from getting loosened. It is often used in cosmetic surgery. It is now more popular in keyhole and laparoscopic surgery.

*Uses of nonabsorbable suture materials:*
- In herniorrhaphy for repair
- For closure of abdomen after laparotomy
- For vascular anastomosis (6-0), nerve suturing, tendon suturing
- In tuboplasty, vasovasostomy—8-0 to 10-0 are used
- In ophthalmic surgeries
- For tension suturing in the abdomen
- For suturing the skin
- In pancreaticojejunostomy

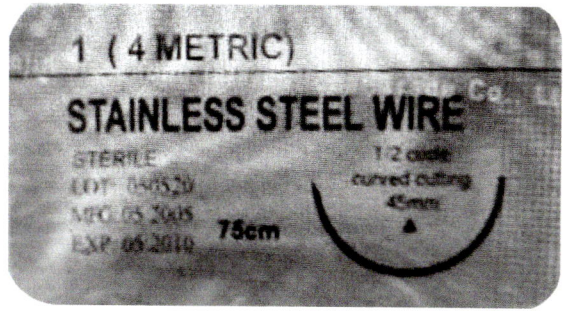

**Fig. 7:** Steel wire is multifilament steel.

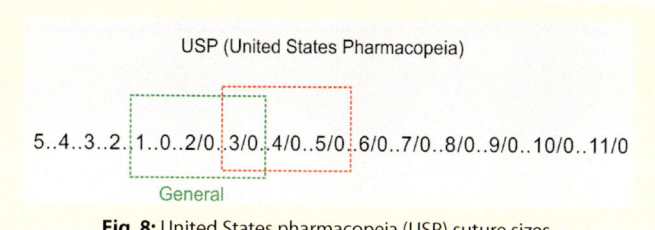

**Fig. 8:** United States pharmacopeia (USP) suture sizes.

## Selection of the Suture Material (Figs. 9 and 10)

It depends on the anatomical location of the wound, type of the wound, tension on the wound and presence of inflammation.

- Scalp—2-0
- Face—4-0 or 5-0
- Lip—5-0
- Eyelid—6-0
- Bowel—3-0
- Tough fascia—2-0 or 1-0 (zero)

Size can be—largest size 2 to extremely fine 11-0. Increasing number of zeroes correlates with decreasing suture diameter and strength. Thicker sutures are used for approximation of deeper layers, wounds in tension prone areas and for ligation of blood vessels. Thin sutures are used for closing delicate tissues like conjunctiva and skin incisions of the face. Size is chosen to correlate with the tensile strength of the tissue being sutured.

## SURGICAL NEEDLES

Surgical needles are devices which penetrate through the tissues to pass sutures across the wounds which are to be approximated. So, needle creates a channel or track to pass the needed suture material with less tissue disruption, with minimum risk of bleeding without compromising the wound blood supply. They are designed to lead suture material through tissue with minimal injury.

*Historically* thorns, ivory, and bone were used as needles and horse hairs were used as sutures. Plant fibers and animal tissues were used as ligatures and sutures in historical days. Later copper and bronze needles were used for suturing. Metal needles became popular in 14th century. Cistercian Monks started eyed needles. Glovemakers straight needle, sailmakers curved needle, handled distal eyelet needle (from gimlet of leather workers) which was used by Pare in 1564 as crooked needles were different needles used in olden days (Fig. 11).

In 1275, Salicet found triangular cutting needle which showed better penetrating property. Mondeville in 1320 started scooping the needle near the eye to accommodate the bulk of the suture material. In 1774, Petit introduced the eyeless concept of the needle where suture material placed in a slot in the needle hub to act like a pincer (Fig. 12). In 1874, Gaillard from San Francisco invented atraumatic needle with its hub end being drilled to place catgut suture which was called as *Eureka needle* (Fig. 13).

Integral flanged needle came in 1921 by Ovington (Davis and Geck Company) (Fig. 14). Now, high-quality stainless steel is used to manufacture needles. Often it is made up of carbon steel. Strength and rigidity are the two important features of a suitable needle. Needle should withstand the optimum force; it may bend but should not break with great force. Needle should have very smooth finish which is created by polishing to clear all burrs on the surface. Needle also should be coated to reduce tissue resistance. But needle often glares to reduce the visibility at the operative field; so, to improve visibility needle is often coated with black chrome (for light bloodless background) or bronze (for reddish blood-filled background).

Surgical needles are made up of stainless steel alloy with 12% chromium and nickel. It is strong and maintains the optimum strength to penetrate the tissues to pass through. Through needles, suture materials are made to pass through the tissues to achieve final strong apposition.

Needle selection is done by the surgeon. It is done based on tissue structure, resistance, thickness, and depth. For soft tissues and skin taper cut needle is sufficient. For tough structures cutting needle is used. Size and body and curvatures are decided depending on the depth and rotation in which needle has to work.

Optimum needle control, optimum needle grip, and optimum needle performance should be achieved; for that, selection of the proper needle holder is important. Needle length, diameter, curvature, and size are important to have a perfect, precised suturing by the surgeon. Force (a measure unit) applied to the needle by the needle holder is *needle holder clamping moment*. *Needle yield moment* is the amount of deformity which can occur before needle is permanently deformed. Needle holder clamping moment must be lesser than needle yield moment.

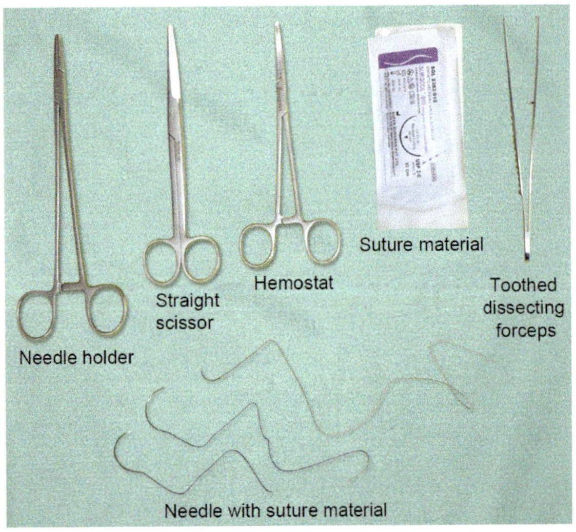

**Fig. 9:** Suturing set.

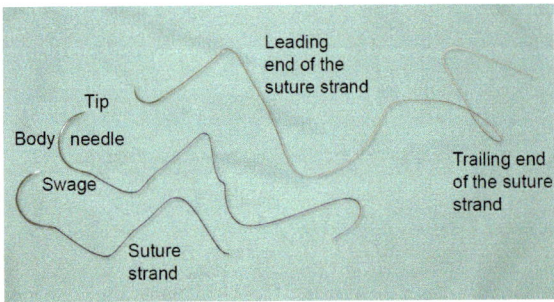

**Fig. 10:** Suture material with needle.

---

*Classification of the surgical needle:*
- *According to eye*—Eyeless needles/Needles with eye.
- *According to shape*—Straight needles/Curved needles.
- *According to cutting edge*—Round body/Cutting—conventional—reverse cutting.
- *According to its tip*—Triangular tip/Round tip/Blunt tip.
- *Others*—Spatula needles/Micropoint needles/Cuticular needles/Plastic needles.

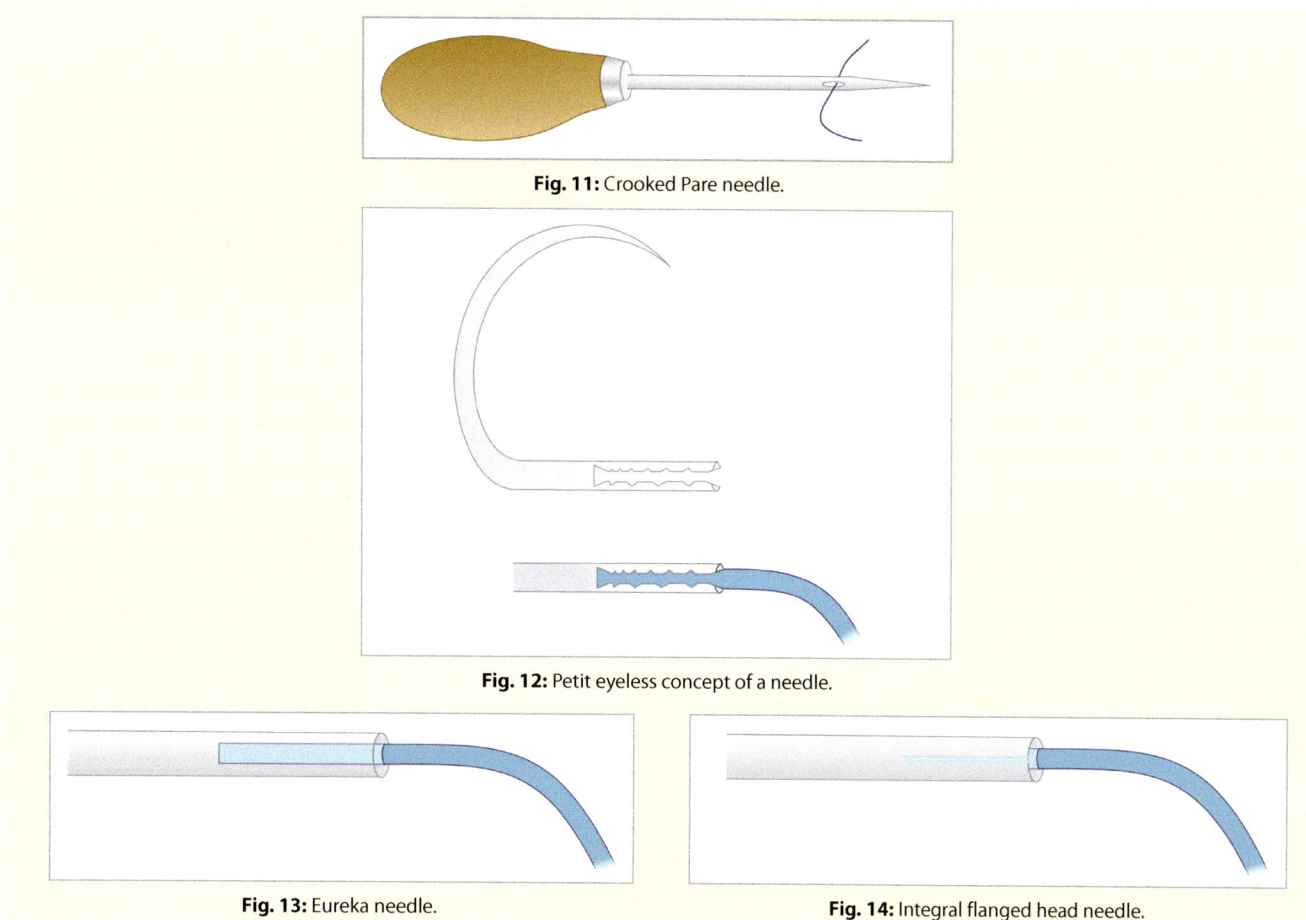

**Fig. 11:** Crooked Pare needle.

**Fig. 12:** Petit eyeless concept of a needle.

**Fig. 13:** Eureka needle.

**Fig. 14:** Integral flanged head needle.

## FEATURES OF SURGICAL NEEDLE

### Needle Integrity

Needle should be strong and should stay firmly in the needle holder (driver) when it is grasped; it should not bend or break during passage through the tissues. Needle rear and tip ends are weak and prone for bend or break. Broken needle may get lost in the tissues or cavities and it is often difficult to identify and remove it; in such situation C—arm imaging may be needed to pinpoint the location of the lost broken needle part. Needle should be rotated along the line and through the tissues needed. It should not be twisted or forced by push. Usually center of the needle is placed at the junction of proximal 2/3rd and distal 1/3rd of the jaw of the needle driver. Integrity and stability of the needle holder should be maintained by the manufacturer.

### Size of the Needle

While selecting the size, both length and diameter of the needle are important for particular suturing. Length is selected depending on the bulk of the tissue being sutured. Diameter of the needle is selected depending on the resistance of the target tissues. Tough structure such as ligaments are sutured using wider stronger cutting needle; smooth tissues such as bowel is sutured using thinner round body needle.

*Length of the needle:* It is essential to select the ideal length of the needle to approximate the given particular tissues. It is selected by assessing the distance between entrance and exit bite points. Wider the distance, lengthier the needle needed. But it is difficult to pass lengthier needle through the tissues as it may get deflected in the needle holder. Withdrawal of the needle is also difficult after holding near its tip.

*Diameter (gauge) of the needle:* Diameter of the needle is equally important in proper suturing technique. Ratio between diameters of needle and suture material is 2 : 1 for larger suture and 3 : 1 for smaller suture even though ideal ratio being 1 : 1 which is not possible to achieve. It is the thickness of the needle; it varies from 30 μ to 1 mm.

*Needle radius:* It is the distance from the center point of the circle of the curvature of the needle (at body).

## PARTS OF A SURGICAL NEEDLE (TABLE 3 AND FIGS. 15A TO C)

It is important to know the different parts of the surgical needle. Types, profiles, and different configurations decide the selection of the needle in different suturing. Operating surgeon should have reasonable idea about the configurations of different types of needles. Important parts are needle tip, body, and swage end.

### Needle Eye

Eye of the needle is the one where suture material is attached to the needle. Eye can

**Table 3:** Description of main components of a needle as well as parts of a surgical needle.

| Parts of a surgical needle: | Main components of a needle: |
|---|---|
| • Needle point is tip<br>• Taper<br>• Shoulder<br>• Body—straight/curved<br>• Eye or suture end<br>• Circumferential length of the needle<br>• Needle chord length—distance between the tip and eye | • *The eye:* The eye can be closed; swaged or chaneled/drilled. Shape of the eye may be round, oblong, or square. Open French-eye needle (Split/spring needle) is easy to load with varying caliber, but has additional bulk<br>• *The body*<br>• *The point (tip)* |

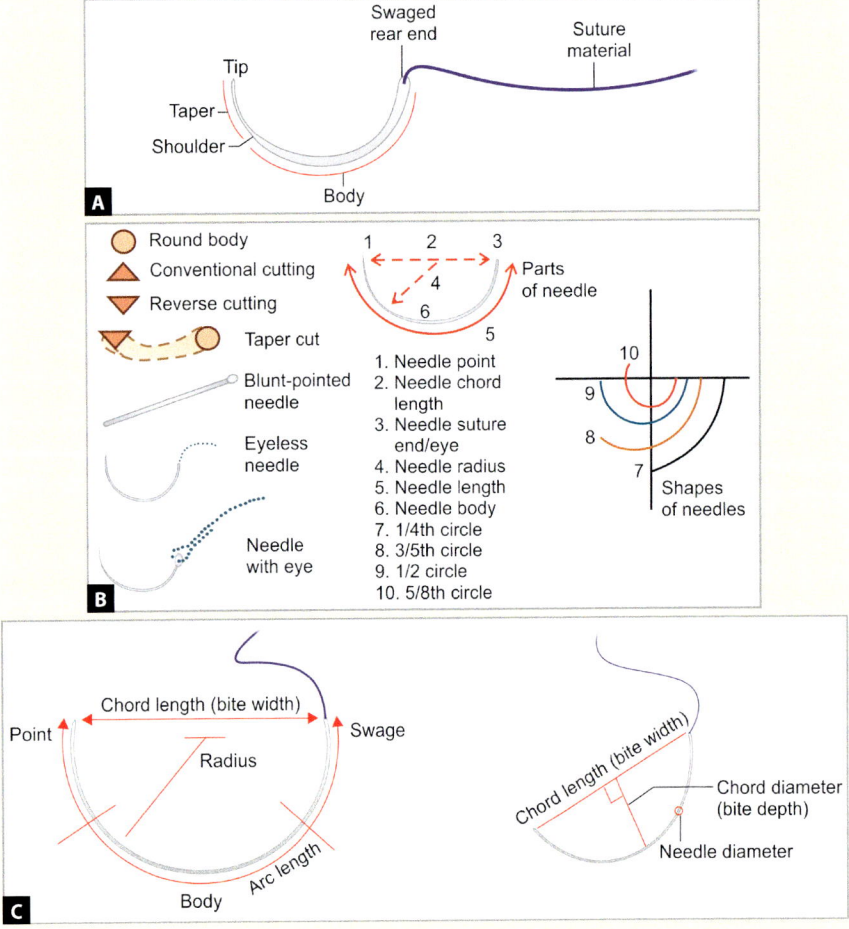

**Figs. 15A to C:** Different parts of the needle. Different types of needles. Diagram also shows the eyeless/eyed needles and gives the meanings of 1/4th, 1/2, 3/8th and 5/8th circle needles.

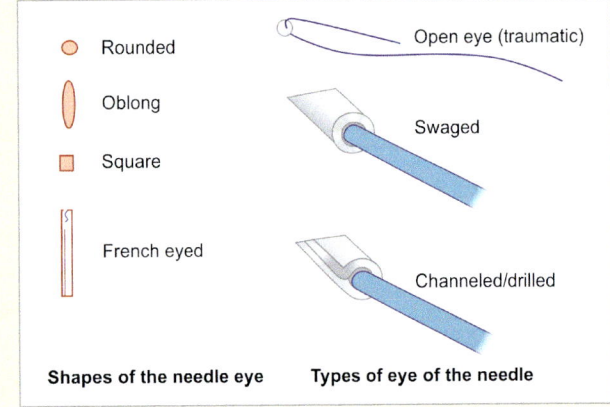

**Fig. 16:** Needle eye types and shapes.

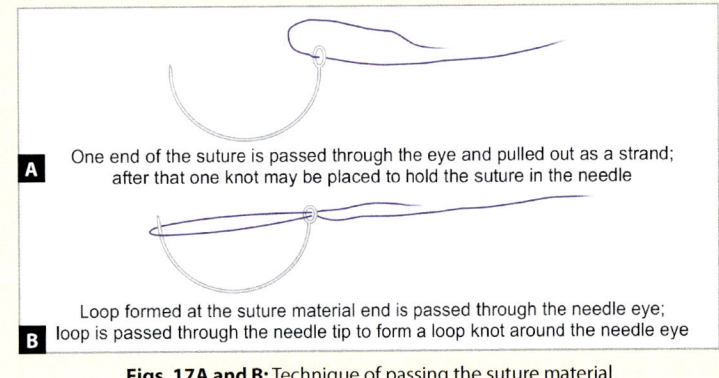

**Figs. 17A and B:** Technique of passing the suture material across the needle eye in open/eyed needle.

be closed (eyelet/eyed needle) or eyeless (atraumatic). Eyeless needle is inbuilt with attached required suture material. It is used only once. Suture material is attached to the needle using different techniques such as—swaging, channeling/drilling/crimping, etc. Attached suture material should be secure and strong; should not get detached from the needle. Eyeless needles with sutures are easy to use; less traumatic to tissues as it is single-stranded. In atraumatic needle, track of the needle and suture material will be same. It is atraumatic and acts as a single unit; prepacked and presterilized. It is manufactured, packed with sterilization either using gamma radiation or ethylene oxide or isopropyl alcohol.

Eyed needles can have different shapes of eye—round/oblong/square **(Fig. 16)**. *French-eyed needle* contains a spring-like action on the eye wherein it is easier to pass the suture material across the eye. Suture is pulled back to create a double-strand (double back). One end is kept shorter than the other by 1/3rd of longer one. Single suture is used for tying. But track will be wider as it has to pass wider eyelet of the needle and two strands of the suture initially. Eyed needles are reusable. It should be sterilized during reuse. Usually chemical sterilization is done. Eyed needle requires threading prior to use, results in pulling a double-strand through tissue. Tying the suture to the eye increases bulk of suture material drawn through tissues. So, they are also called *"traumatic needles"*. Suture material end is passed through the needle eye and pulled out using a forceps or hemostat and often one knot is placed to keep the suture material in place. Alternatively, loop of the suture material end is passed through the needle eye and is looped around the needle tip to reach the eye as a slip knot **(Figs. 17A and B)**.

### Different Techniques to Attach the Needle to Suture Material in Atraumatic Eyeless Needle

*Swaging:* Rear end of the needle is first flattened **(Fig. 18)**; it is folded to create a U-shaped channel; the suture is kept in this groove and metal is folded around the channel to grip the suture end using a precise force to achieve security. Diameter is reconstituted and burrs are eliminated. Here double strands of a suture material are eliminated. It also allows the placement of needle on both ends of a suture material to create a *double-armed suture* **(Fig. 19)**. One should remember the swaging junction is the *weakest point of a suture material*.

*Crimping:* Using mechanical device or laser, a tunnel is drilled at the rear end of the needle. End of the suture material is inserted into the tunnel. It is crimped in place securely using optimum force. Crimping is used for a larger diameter suture **(Fig. 20)**.

*Metalized suture:* It is done to eliminate weak point created either by swaging or crimping. Electroplating and dipping was tried to attach the suture. But it is not in common usage.

### Needle Body

Body of the needle is the part proximal to the shoulder or proximal to taper. Body extends up to the rear end that is swage. It may be rounded or oval (currently popular) or triangular or reverse cut or flattened hexagonal or rhomboid or diamond-shaped on cross-section **(Figs. 21A and B)**. Body may be having grooves or ribs on the inner and outer surfaces of the body. Body may be straight or curved. Needle is held in this part using needle holder either middle or distal 1/3rd (needle arming). Body is the widest portion of the needle; it is known as grasping area. Most commonly used are 3/8 circle. They can easily be manipulated in large and superficial wounds and require only less wrist movement. 1/2 circle is used for suturing tissues in small wounds, and body cavities and orifices. It requires less space, but more supination and pronation of wrist is required. 5/8 circle is used in oral cavity.

Curved needle is commonly used. This curve is used with a dynamic driving force using needle driver to penetrate through the tissues effectively and efficiently. Shape, size, dimension of the curvature, strength, and stability of needle are important to have an optimum safe and efficient needle. Needle should be grasped properly by the needle holder; this grasp efficiency prevents the needle from deflecting and moving in the jaws of the needle holder. Needle should be strong enough to pass through the tissues required without bending or breaking. It should be easily penetrable and should withstand the force used to pass the needle.

### Shoulder of the Needle

It is the junction of the body and taper of a needle. Configurations will be different on either sides of the shoulder. Needle driver (holder) is placed in the body just proximal to the shoulder.

### Needle Tip

Distal most part of the needle is needle tip. It is the one which allows the penetration of the needle through the tissues efficiently. Tip is sharp enough to penetrate the tissues. Easy penetration depends on tapering ratio,

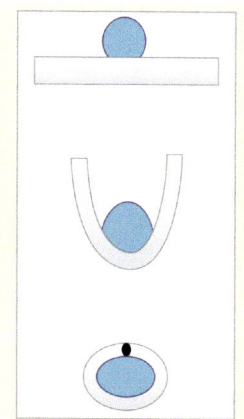

**Fig. 18:** Swaging of the needle to the suture material—rear end is flattened; then folded to create a U; suture is placed into the groove of created U and arms of the U is folded to create strong "O" with suture material end captured inside.

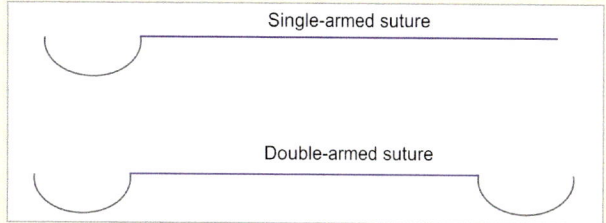

**Fig. 19:** Single-armed and double-armed sutures. Here similar needles are attached on both ends of the suture.

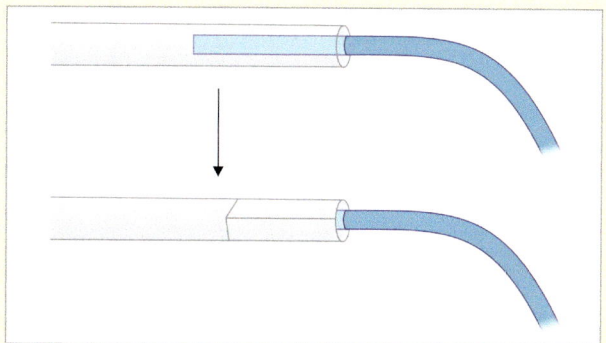

**Fig. 20:** Crimping method.

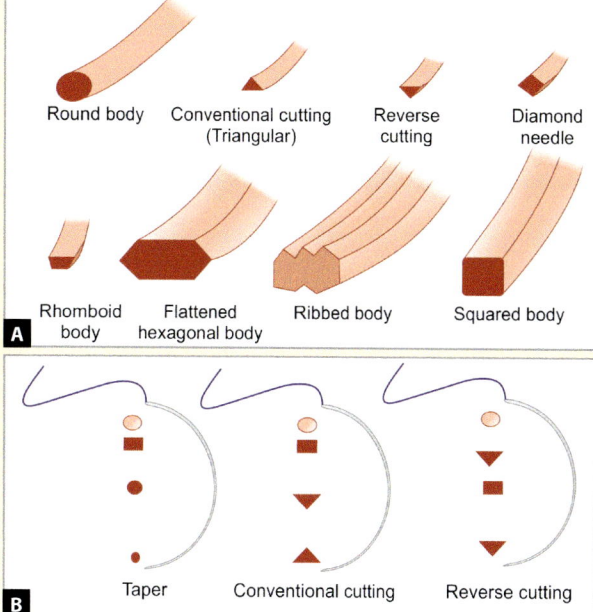

**Figs. 21A and B:** Different types of the body of the needle. Round body, conventional cutting, and reverse cutting are different types.

cross-section of the needle. Blunt needle tip is used in infected cases to avoid possible injury to the operating team. It can be triangular tip/cutting or round tip or blunt tip. The conventional cutting point has two opposing cutting edges and third edge on the inside curvature of the needle. The reverse cutting point has two opposing cutting edges and third cutting edge on the outer curvature of the needle.

### Tapering of the Needle

Needle tapers up to the shoulder of the needle but tapering distance varies. Tapering ratio is the ratio between distance, between the needle point and shoulder of the needle, and diameter at body of the needle **(Fig. 22)**. If tapering length is 8 mm and diameter at body is 2 mm then tapering ratio is 4:1. Usually 3:1 tapering ratio is commonly used. More the tapering the ratio better the penetration capacity; but needle is prone for bending and loss of strength. Tapering tip may be cutting or round-bodied (noncutting). Round-bodied taper tip is used in vascular and bowel anastomosis to achieve minimum trauma in the tissue track. Cutting tip is used for skin and tough structures. Cutting tip may be conventional triangular (Δ) or reverse cutting (∇). Spatulated tip is also useful in tough structures such as cornea, periosteum, and ligaments. Here tip (apex) is triangular or reverse and proximally taper up to the shoulder of the needle as rhomboid spatulated again either as conventional or inverse spatula **(Figs. 23A and B)**.

> **Features of an ideal surgical needle:**
> - It is made up of high quality stainless needle.
> - It should be stable to be grasped by the jaws of the needle driver.
> - It should be adequately sharp enough to penetrate the required tissue.
> - It should be sterile and corrosive resistant.
> - Smaller diameter is ideal to minimize the tissue trauma.
> - *Strength* (resistance to deformation during passage through tissues); *ductility* (resistance to breakage after bending); *sharpness* (ability to penetrate the tissues easily); and *clamping moment* (stability of the needle in a needle driver) are different qualities/characteristics which decide the needle performance.

### Types

#### Based on the Edge

- *Round body needle:* It is round and smooth on cross-section. It is used to suture muscles/intestines/soft tissues/vessels/nerves/tendons/peritoneum.
- *Taper round needle:* Round-bodied needle tapering smoothly toward the tip. Tapering ratio and tip angle (20–35°) decide the sharpness (high taper with low tip angle). It is useful in subcutaneous tissue, dura, mucosa, bowel, fascia, etc.
- *Conventional cutting needle:* Here needle is triangular on cross-section with apex facing inward. It is used to suture skin/aponeurosis/tough structures. Cutting edge is inside the curve. Needle has got three edges; initial triangular cross-section area; next flat area; end triangular cutting with cutting point on the inner concave side (surface seeking).
- *Reverse cutting needle:* Here needle is triangular (reverse) on cross-section with apex facing outward. It increases the strength and is less likely to bend while suturing. Here cutting edge is outside the curve. Reverse cutting needle is stronger than conventional cutting needle (depth seeking). It is used in mucoperiosteum, tendon, skin or tough structure.
- *Taper cut needle:* Here tip of the needle is cutting or reverse cutting in section but eventually tapers into the body as round in section. It improves the penetration of needle but minimizes the trauma.
- Blunt pointed needles are used to suture friable organs such as liver/spleen/kidneys.
- *Spatulated side cutting needle* (saber lock)—is like a spatula with two lateral side cutting edges; used in ophthalmic surgeries.
- *Micropoint needles,* either round bodied or reverse cutting or spatulated, are used in ophthalmic surgery and microsurgery. It has got an extra honing process.

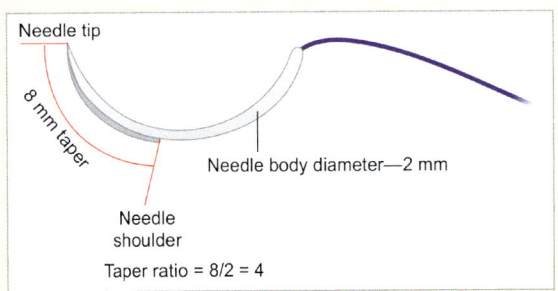

**Fig. 22:** Tapering ratio of the needle is the ratio between distance, between the needle point and shoulder of the needle, and diameter at body of the needle.

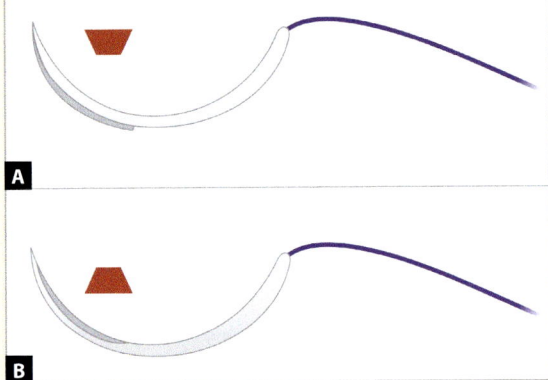

**Figs. 23A and B:** Spatulated needle tips. (A) Conventional spatulated; (B) Inverse spatulated.

- *Trocar point needle* is stout strong cutting end with a robust round body. It is used in obstetrics and gynecology.
- *Tru taper needle* is one with tip angle of needle is at 22° (unlike conventional angle is 32°). It is used in vascular surgery.
- *Visiblack needles*—Needles coated with black so that they are visible better in red background. It also prevents the glare from the focus lights by the needles.
- *Dolphin nose needle* is especially designed needle used for surgeries in patients with hepatitis and AIDS which minimizes the risk of puncturing the gloves and fingers of the surgeon.
- *JB needle* (Juergen–Breunner needle)— oval round-bodied needle with a steep curve at the distal half to have easy passage of the needle through bowel in gastrointestinal surgeries.
- *Port closure needle* in laparoscopic surgeries.
- *Ski needle* with a ski-shaped curvature in the distal part so as to have easy passage through the port for laparoscopic intra-corporeal suturing **(Figs. 24 and 25)**.
- *Cuticular needles:* It is sharpened 12 times; designated as C or FS (Cuticular or For Skin).
- *Plastic needles:* It is sharpened an additional 24 times; designated as P or PS or PC (Premium or Plastic Surgery or Precision Cosmetic); needles in the PC series are made up of stronger SS alloy and have flattened and conventional cutting edge.

### Based on Curvature

- *Straight needle:* It was once commonly used needle (*Keith needle for skin and Bunnel needle for GIT*). It can be cutting or round bodied. It too can be with eyelet or atraumatic. Atraumatic straight round body needles with chromic catgut suture were popular in olden days while doing bowel anastomosis. Straight needle is still often used for skin suturing especially by beginners; it is quiet useful in laparoscopic surgery also.
- *Curved needle:* 1/4, 1/2, 3/8, and 5/8 circle, etc. 1/2 and 3/8 are commonly used. It is the wrist movement which rotates the needle through tissues. Surgeons often reconfigure the needle to their personal preference. While bending the needle to needed movement, needle at the point of bent gets weakened and may break. Needle holder should not be used to reshape the needle as carbide jaw of the needle may blur the surface of the needle making it more traumatic.
- *Compound needles:* Here configurations at the tip and body are different. J-shaped needle, fishhook needle, and compound curved needles are different types which are self-explanatory. They are used in depth to have controlled penetration of the needle during suturing—suturing in depth in the pelvis, in ophthalmology procedures.
- *Endoski needle* **(Figs. 26A and B)**: This needle is especially devised for laparoscopic surgery. Here proximal component of the needle is straight with distal dynamic part is curved as half of a half-circle; straight component is one-and-half trims of the curved one. The shaft is either triangular or rhomboid. Triangular type avoids both swivel and deflection of the needle. Rhomboid type resists swivel. Curved part is tapered. Needle can be passed through 5-mm port easily into the peritoneal cavity. Needle is held using laparoscopic needle holder along the straight component. But while driving the needle, direction of the dynamic end needle tip is difficult to make out, so that any deflection, if occurs, cannot be identified easily.

### Based on Existence of the Eye

- *Atraumatic needle* is eyeless. Here suture material is attached to the needle by *swaging* (Mr Merson of England). Size of the suture material and that of needle is same or less and so tissue trauma is less. It is single-stranded. Needle once used is disposed. (Not reusable).

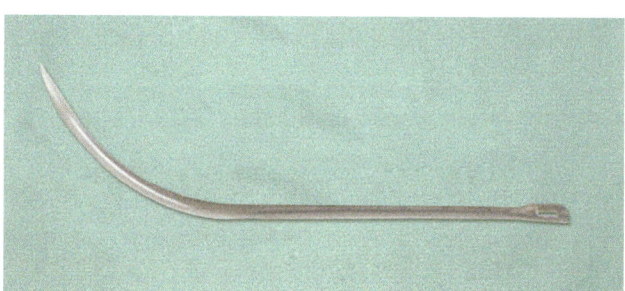

**Fig. 24:** Ski needle.

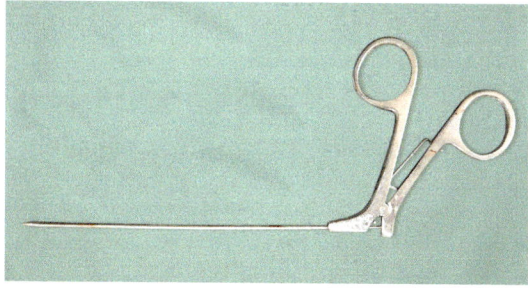

**Fig. 25:** Laparoscopic port closure needle.

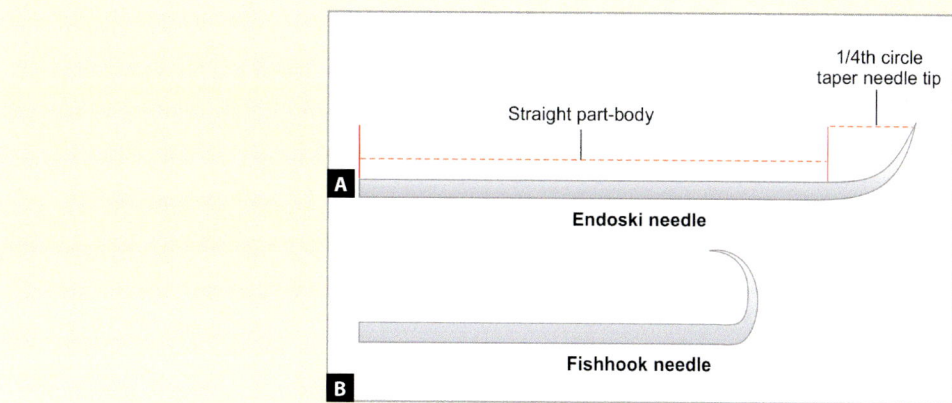

**Figs. 26A and B:** (A) Endoski needle is commonly used in laparoscopy; (B) Fishhook needle used in depth.

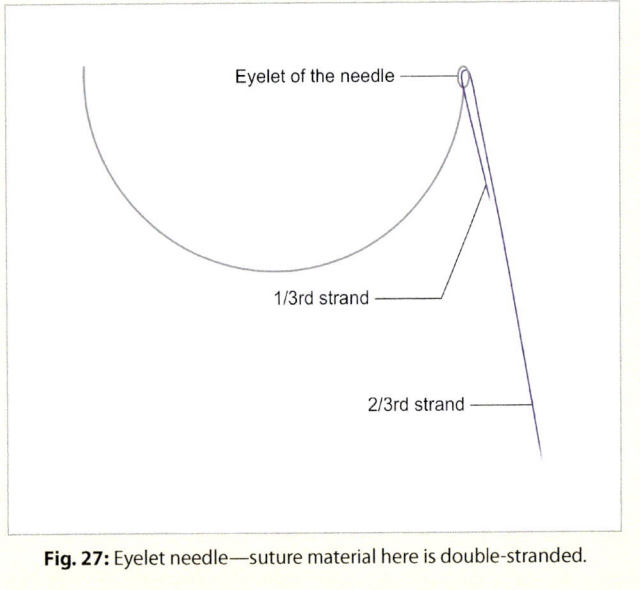

**Fig. 27:** Eyelet needle—suture material here is double-stranded.

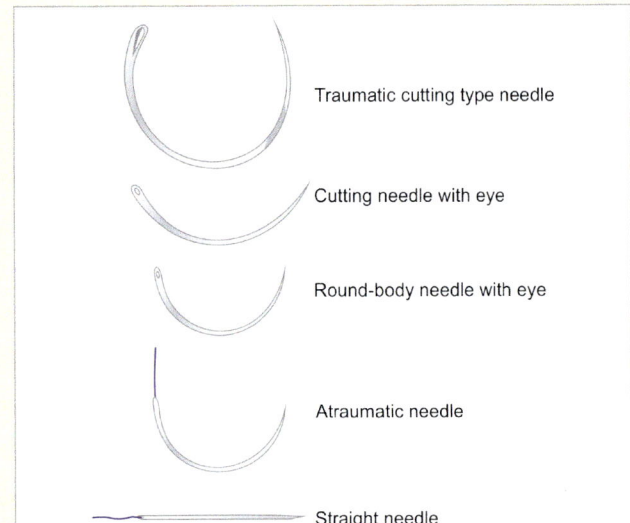

**Fig. 28:** Different types of needles.

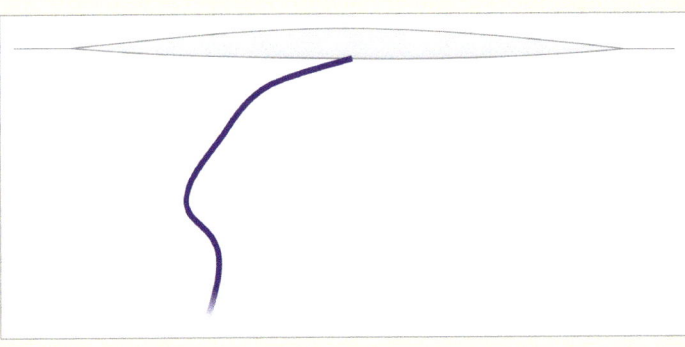

**Fig. 29:** Shuttle needle.

It is available as sterilized pack. These needles can be round body or cutting. As it is single use needle, patient develops a new guaranteed sharp sterile needle. Accidental unthreading is not present. High-quality efficacy of the needle is present, so suturing is easier, quicker, and better.

- *Traumatic needle:* It is eyed needle (French eyelet—14th century) **(Figs. 27 and 28)**. Needle in the eye area is wider than the body of the needle and so tissue trauma is more. These needles are re-usable. It should be sterilized prior to reuse. Accidental fall of thread or needle may be problematic here.
- *Half-curved needles at both ends of a straight part (Canoe needle).*

*Note:*
- The weakest part of the needle is part near the eye.
- Needle is sterilized in cidex/lysol. It should not be autoclaved as tip gets blunt.
- The needle is held at its center by placing it at the junction of the proximal 2/3rd and distal 1/3rd to have optimal grip, control and precision.
- Needles can be 1/4 circle, 1/2 circle, 3/8 circle or 5/8 circle at their curvatures. (Refer diagram for the same). Needles of different curvature are used at different places depending on the depth of the suturing.
- Needles are made up of stainless steel.
- Atraumatic needles are available as sterilized packs. They are sterilized by ethylene oxide or gamma sterilization along with the sutures which they coexist.
- *Gallie's needle* is large eyed needle which was earlier used in hernias to suture the defect using fascia lata strips.
- *Lane's needle* is half-circle cutting needle with a large eye.
- *Mayo needle* is obstetric needle with a large square eye and is strong.
- *Hagedorn reverse flattened point fishhook needle* used for suturing inaccessible sites.
- *Symonds round bodied fishhook needles.*
- *Bonney Reverdin needle* is a special needle with an eye which is open to one side with small slender shutter which can be slid and closed after passing the suture material.
- *Kousnetzoff aluminum needle is* used to suture the liver tear.

## SHUTTLE NEEDLE

Usually suture material is attached to the *end of the needle*. But in *middle attachment needle (shuttle needle)* suture material is attached to the middle of a straight needle **(Fig. 29)**. It is useful in laparoscopic surgery but otherwise causes double track in the tissue passage. *Detachable suture material* is often used where purposefully suture material is attached to needle with a low force so that after passage through the tissue needle can be detached from the suture material with reasonable distraction force on the suture and needle in opposite directions. It is useful in some open surgeries but should not be used in laparoscopic surgeries. Chances of needle getting missed in the surgical field are higher when such needles are used.

# CHAPTER 4

# Principles of Suturing

*"It is the supreme art of the teacher to awaken joy in creative expression and knowledge"*
*"A teacher affects eternity he can never tell where his influence" stops.*

–Henry Adams

## INTRODUCTION

Suturing technique is similar in most places; even then selection of ideal needle driver (holder), needle size, type, suture material—type, number (size) makes suturing easier, artistic and perfect. Tension free, adequate depth, perfect alignment, proper eversion without causing compromised blood supply of the wound edges are essential technical precautions that should be taken. The basic purpose of a suture is to hold disrupted tissues in close approximation until the healing process provides the wound sufficient strength to withstand stress. Suture material should be at least as strong as the tissues in which they are used. Wound will regain its tensile strength only up to 80% of its original strength, not more than that.

## PRINCIPLES

It is essential to avoid damage to suture strand when handling. One should touch strands only with gloved hand or closed blunt instrument. One should not crush or crimp sutures with instruments except when grasping the suture during instrument tie. Suture material should not be held using needle holder or artery forceps except during knotting.

*Goals of wound closure are* no infection, normal function, and optimum/excellent cosmesis. These goals are achieved by minimal bacterial contamination; removal of the devitalized tissues with foreign bodies; proper hemostasis; gentle tissue-handling using forceps (skin-toothed forceps, soft tissues non-toothed fine forceps); optimum approximation of tissues only but not strangulation. *Forceps should be held between thumb and middle finger with index finger being used for stabilization* **(Fig. 1)**.

Proper selection of the needle holder, type of needles (size, curve, etc.), and suture material is important. Needle is placed in the needle holder at the junction of *proximal 2/3rd to distal 1/3rd* of the jaws of needle holder to have optimum grip and precision. If held more proximal, then grip

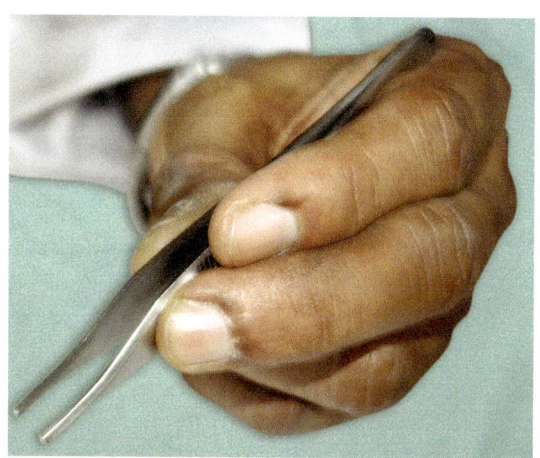

**Fig. 1:** Forceps should be held between thumb and middle finger with index finger being used for stabilization.

will be good but precision is inadequate. If needle is more distally placed, precision is good but with poor grip. Needle is held *half the distance from swaged end*. Grasping of the needle should be neither too tight nor too loose. Usually, one ratchet catch in the needle holder is sufficient to have optimum grip; excessive tightening should be avoided to prevent damaging both needle and needle holder **(Fig. 2)**. Optimum *grasp* should be there. Alignment of the jaws of needle holder should be proper. Needle should not rotate during grasping. Needle and needle holder should function as a *single unit*. Different needle holders are available such as Olsen Hegar needle holder, Kilner needle holder, Mayo Hager needle, and Yasargil micro needle holder **(Figs. 3 to 5)**. Gripping the needle holder is important. The scissor grip is used in the anterior part of the mouth and in areas of easy access; the instrument is stabilized with the index finger. Palm grip is used in the deeper parts of oral cavity or in depth.

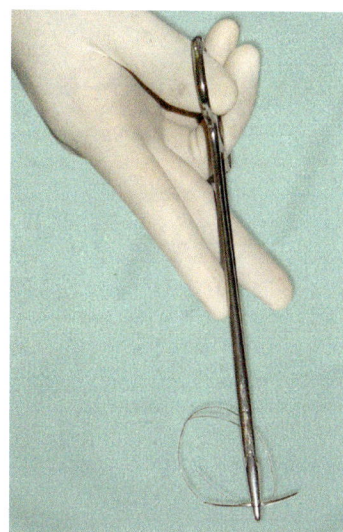

**Fig. 2:** Holding the needle in a needle holder. Holding the needle holder properly and knowing its movement in rotational axis is important for proper suturing and knotting. It is the precise gentle rotation which is essential; not pushing flimsy movement.

- Appropriate sized needle holder for the respective needle should be used.
- Needle should be grasped 1/2 to 2/3rd distance from swaged area.
- Tips of the jaws should meet before remaining portion of jaw.
- Needle should be placed securely.
- Needle holder should be locked while using but should not be overclosed.
- Needle holder should always be directed by surgeon's thumb.
- Rotation movement should be used.
- Optimum grip and optimum control are needed for precise work.
- Stability and dexterity are important.

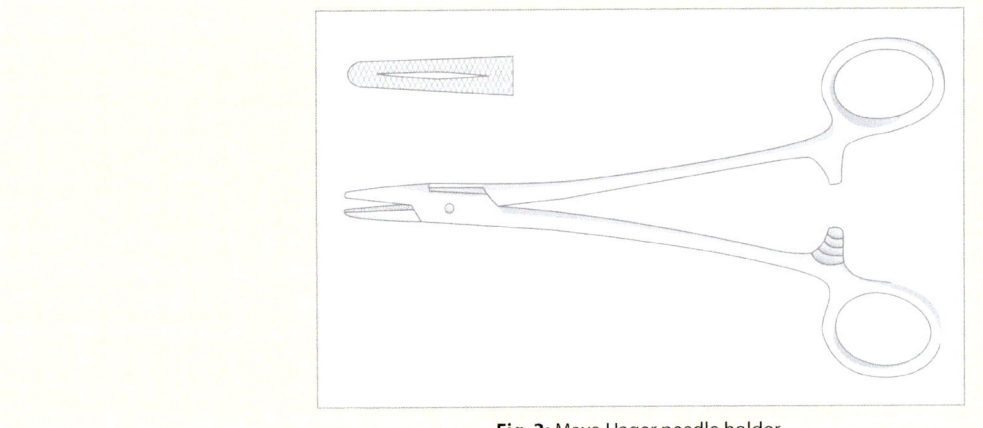

**Fig. 3:** Mayo Hager needle holder.

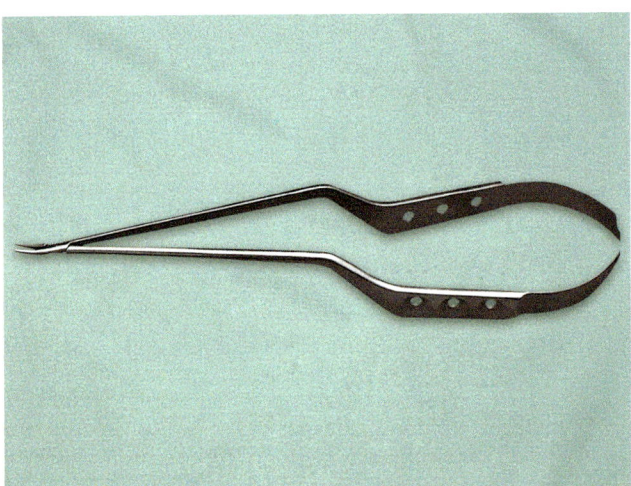

**Fig. 4:** Yasargil micro needle holder.

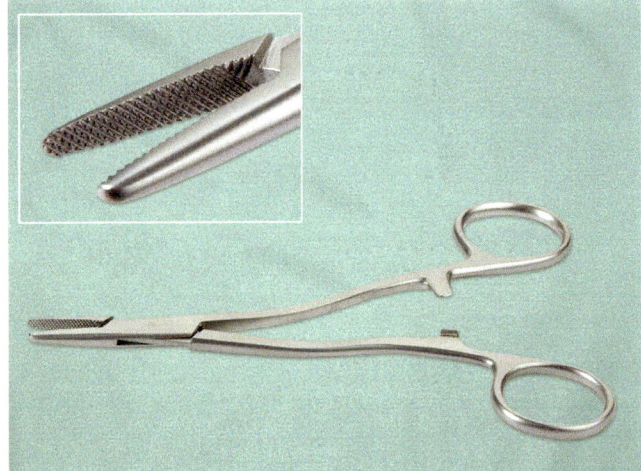

**Fig. 5:** Kilner needle holder.

*The choice of suture* for a particular procedure is based on the known physical and biologic characteristics of the suture material and the healing properties of the sutured tissues. It also depends on condition of the disrupted tissues and condition of the patient and postoperative status. In potentially contaminated areas, monofilament sutures are better (like polypropylene). When cosmetic result is anticipated, fine inert monofilament sutures are used.

*In vascular suturing*, monofilament polypropylene is used which is inert, least infective, least reactive, with high tensile strength, and least thrombus formation. Size selection depends on the size of the vessel and situation, where it is being used 4-0 to 7-0 are used. Polyester is preferred for suturing artificial heart valves, myocardium, and vascular prosthesis.

*In irradiated field*, not only the normal healing process is delayed but the tolerance to the trauma of irradiated tissue is markedly reduced. Extreme careful and gentle surgical technique is needed and sutures with tension should be avoided as they further increase the degree of ischemia. Nonabsorbable polypropylene or polyglactin absorbable can be used. Intermittent sutures are ideal than continuous one.

*In microsurgical procedure*, polyamide or polypropylene 10-0 is used.

When a wound has reached maximal strength, then sutures are no longer needed. Tissues that ordinarily heal slowly such as skin, fascia, and tendons should be sutured with nonabsorbable sutures. Tissues that heal rapidly such as peritoneum, liver, small intestine, muscles, stomach, colon, and bladder are sutured with absorbable sutures; but in gastrointestinal tract, nonabsorbable sutures are also used. Suture should be stronger than the sutured tissues. It is not good to use more suture material than necessarily needed to avoid adverse problems such as crumpling and tissue strangulation.

*The selection of suture material is based on:*
- The condition of the wound
- The tissues to be repaired
- The tensile strength of the suture material
- Knot-holding characteristics of the suture material
- The reaction of surrounding tissues to the suture materials.

Forward wrist movement (*fluid movement of the wrist*) and back-hand movement are important movements in suturing. Mainly wrist and partly elbow movements are used in combination. Shoulder movements should be restricted as much as possible. Height of the table and stance of the surgeon and changing stance as per need are equally important for effective suturing.

*Correct placement of the needle* (*Needle arming*) is essential to have proper easy penetration of the tissue at desired angle. Needle should be held in the middle of the needle in the body using needle holder; needle is placed at the distal jaw of the needle holder at the junction of distal 1/3rd and proximal 2/3rd; and the needle holder should be locked adequately. Usually, needle holder (driver) is held using thumb and fourth finger and index finger rests on the fulcrum of the needle holder to create stability **(Figs. 6A to C)**. Often needle holder can be held in the palm to increase the dexterity.

Tissue to be penetrated by needle should be held using dissecting forceps. For skin and tough structures, toothed forceps

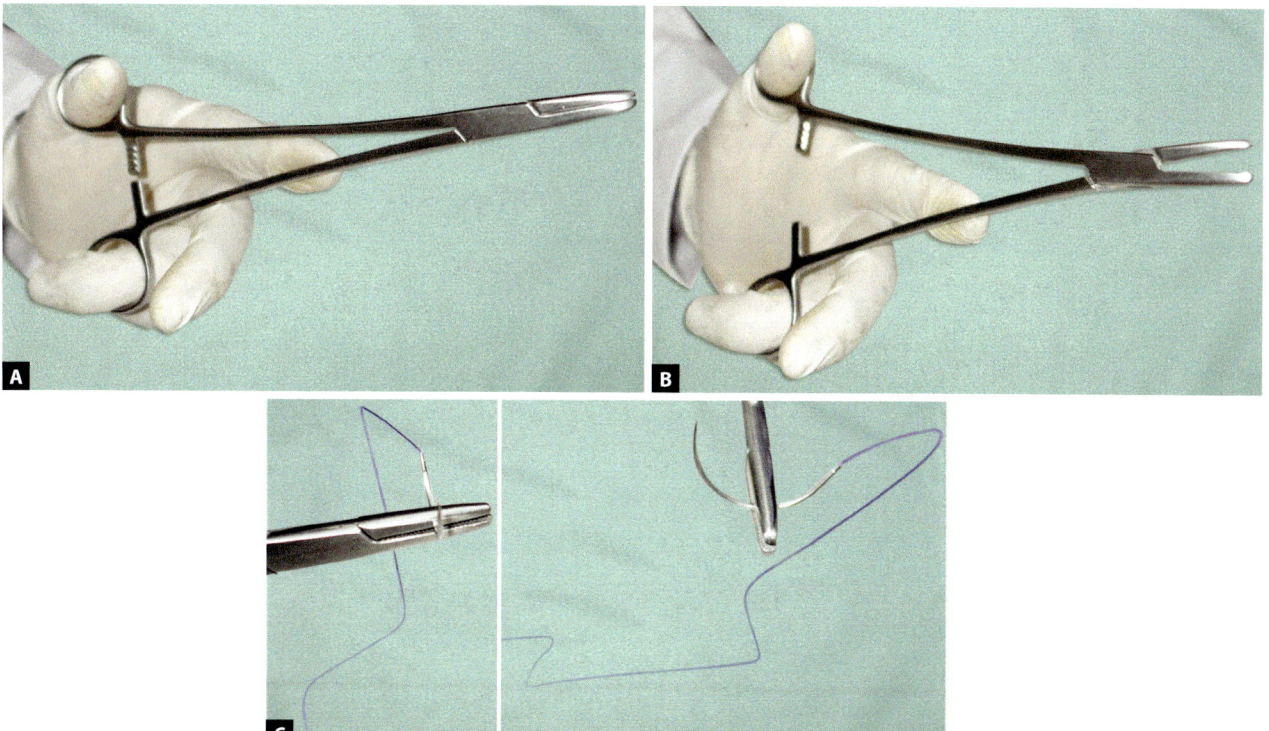

**Figs. 6A to C:** Holding needle holder in different ways.

are used; for bowel, soft tissues, muscles, vessels, peritoneum, etc. are held using non-toothed forceps. Often finer forceps such as Adson's forceps are used. Undue traction on the tissue should not be done as it may traumatize or tear the tissues. If tissues are in depth or bulky instead of taking bites together from the wound edges, it is preferable to take bites one after another from each edge of the wound so that precision in taking the adequate tissue bite with alignment becomes perfect.

Needle should enter the tissue/skin *perpendicular to the surface at 90° allowing smooth entry* without any tissue damage; similarly needle should exit out through exit tissue also at 90°. Width, depth at entry point, and exit points should become near mirror image of each other. *While bringing out of the exit tissue, needle (body) proximal to the tip should be held with forceps ideally even though it is done using needle holder especially in deeper tissues. Needle tip should not be held as repetitive friction will blunt or dull the needle tip or tip may rarely break also.* Coordinated use of forceps and needle driver with alternating pronating and supinating hand actions with needle holder is important to achieve effective and efficient least traumatic suture placement and creating a rectangular suture path **(Figs. 7A to C)**.

Needle is passed through smaller thickness of the tissue. Excess tissue bite should be avoided. It is the smooth, rotation movement than the movement with force which is important. Proper sized needle should be taken depending on the thickness and texture of tissue/tissue resistance, which is to be apposed. *Rotation force should be in the direction of the curvature of needle. Twisting or bending needle tip should be avoided. Holding the needle tip with instrument will cause blunting or breaking of the tip and if such broken tip is entangled in the tissue it is very difficult to identify it.*

While suturing, after taking the proper needle bite through one edge of the wound (skin or tissues), needle holder is released but forceps should hold the tissue/skin edge until needle holder is completely released and adequate length of the needle tip is visible; then forceps is released from the tissue and needle is grasped using forceps to place it in the needle holder again. Needle is again similarly pierced from inside outside to complete the suturing; again here also needle tip should be adequately pierced and visible to hold the needle tip with forceps; entire act of suturing requires proper fine pronation and supination of the wrist. Bites from both the edges of the wound can be taken together without releasing the needle from the needle holder but forceps is released from first edge to hold the second edge while taking respective needle bites. It is done in surface wounds; but while suturing in the depth or whenever difficulty arises it is ideal to take bites from each edge separately so that proper bite is ensured **(Figs. 8A and B)**. Needle should pierce 5 mm from the wound edge in general but perpendicular to the tissue, i.e., equidistant from the both cut edges.

*In a lengthy wound,* first suture is placed at the center of the wound; next one middle of this center sutured part to the end of the wound; next one to opposite end similarly in its center; later remaining sutures are placed. This allows the proper alignment of the wound closure without any overlapping **(Figs. 9A to C)**.

*Cutting needles* are used for skin, tough structures, and mucoperiosteum. *Round bodied needles* are used for smooth tissues such as fat, peritoneum, muscle, bowel, vessel anastomosis, etc. Usual *width of the tissue* taken is 5 mm. But, finally, it depends on the thickness, tissue strength, and condition to which patient is getting operated upon. In retention sutures of abdomen or Smead–Jones closure, width taken is 3 cm. Distance between each bite is important. It should not be too close nor too far. In the skin, 1 cm gap between sutures is sufficient. In the bowel 5-mm gap between sutures is needed to have complete sealing of the bowel edge and also hemostasis. Tissue should be handled carefully. Only the tissue that is required should be grasped. Bulk grasping should be avoided. Smaller-sized suture is better.

*Size of the suture material* is decided in relation to the strength of the tissues. Usually, 3-0 is used. Thicker tissues may need 2-0 sutures. Abdominal wall closure needs 1 or 0 or 1-0 suture material.

Ideally, interrupted sutures are better. It holds and apposes well. It maintains the blood supply of the tissue edge. But in many places such as gastrojejunostomy continuous sutures can be used.

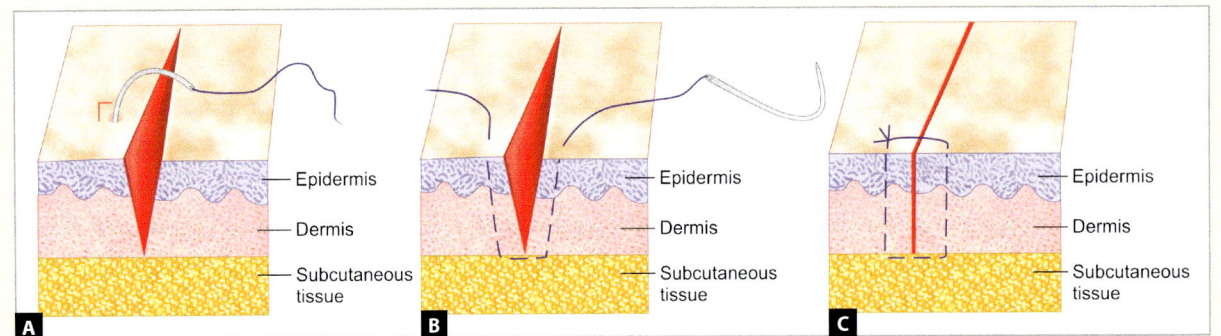

**Figs. 7A to C:** Principles shown in simple interrupted suture placement. (A) Needle should pierce the skin/tissue perpendicular to the surface; (B) From equidistant opposite side, needle should come out after deep full thickness bite; (C) Final knot towards one side (not on the wound edge) with proper apposition without dead space.

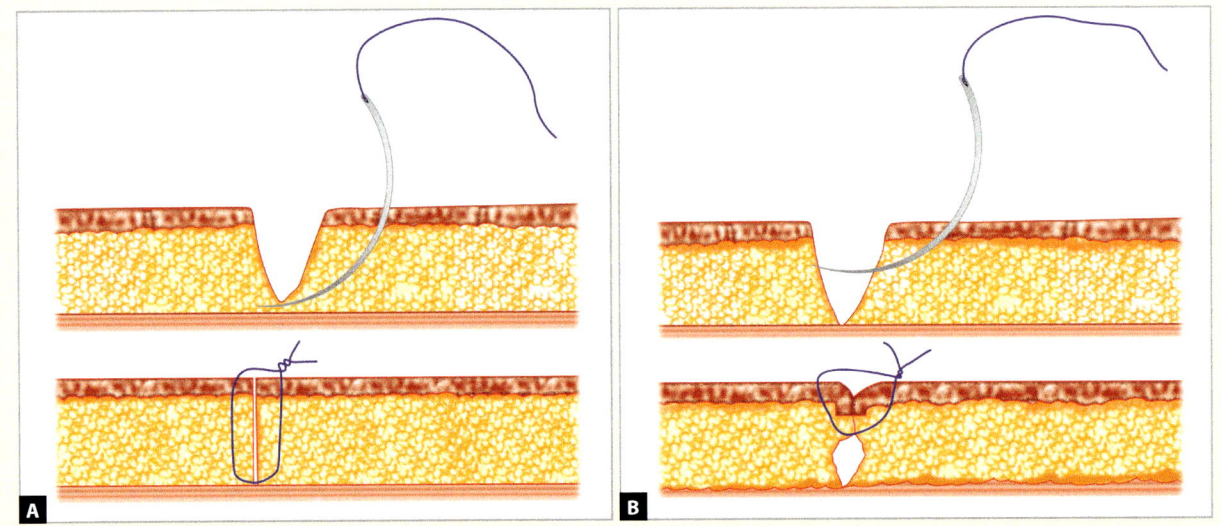

**Figs. 8A and B:** (A) While suturing needle bite should be correctly with adequate depth. Deeper part should be wider than to have proper apposition; (B) Taking wrong bite of needle with inadequate depth, width and inequality will cause poor apposition and alignment and also creating dead space in the deeper plane causing seroma formation or poor scar later.

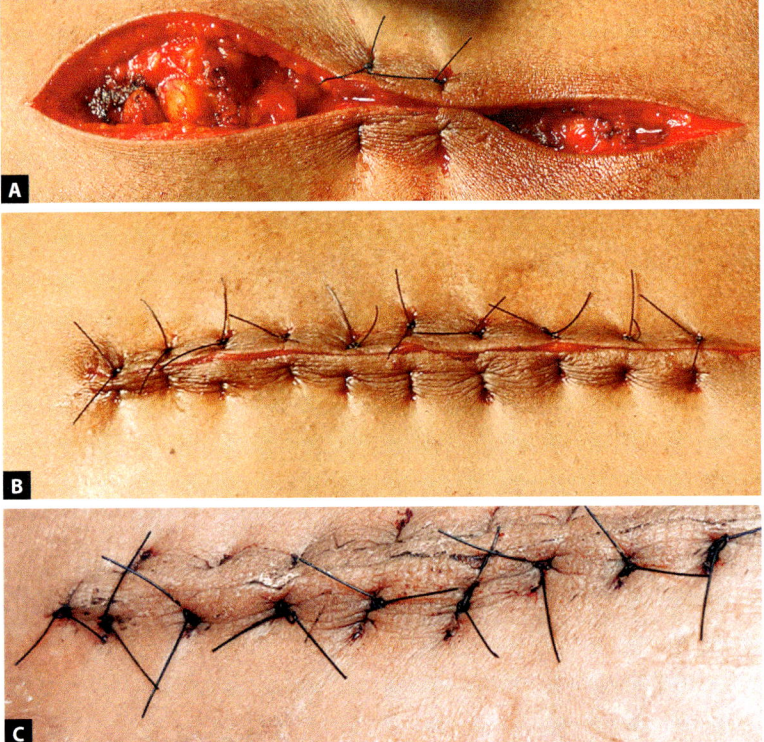

**Figs. 9A to C:** Technique of suturing the lengthy wound to achieve proper alignment without overlapping.

It is better to take bite from each edge of the tissue *separately* even though it looks more time consuming. When both edges are held together and needle is forced through them, there are chances of having lateral movements which can cause tear at the first point of entry of the needle resulting in poor apposition of the tissue **(Fig. 10)**. It can be used safely, if the edges are close enough without tension, and if one can avoid lateral movements while taking bite of second edge.

Learner *should practice* holding the tissues with instruments than hand. It is common that beginner prefers to use hands than instruments as it is easier, but holding tissues with instruments is better. In certain occasions, hand is used to hold the tissues; otherwise by enlarge instruments are used. Technique of simple interrupted suture placement with its principles is shown here **(Figs. 11 and 12)**.

*Type of suture material* used depends on the tissue and condition for which suturing is done. Once wound attains maximum strength, sutures are no longer required. Slow healing wounds need nonabsorbable sutures. Rapidly healing wound need

# Principles of Suturing

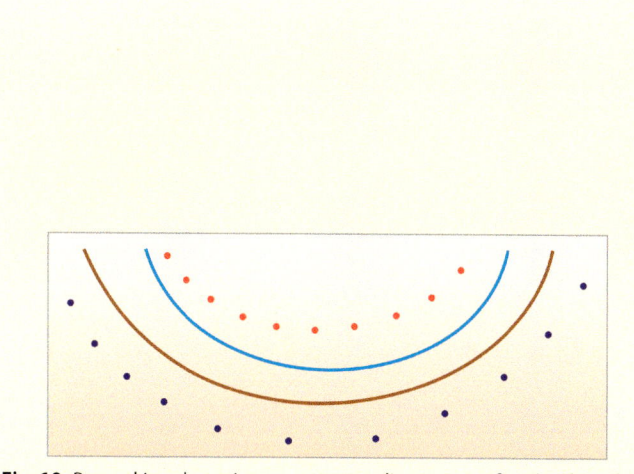

**Fig. 10:** By marking the points at corresponding points of each edge of the wound before suturing, makes it easier to take bites at proper anatomical level to achieve good wound alignment and apposition without causing disparity.

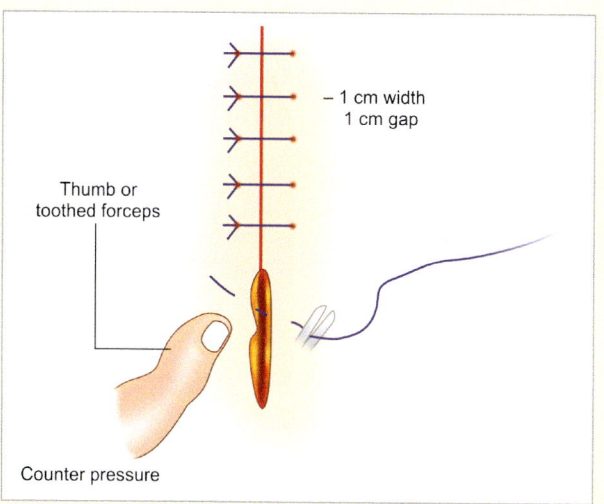

**Fig. 11:** Equidistant, proper correct bite, counter pressure using thumb or toothed forceps on the opposite edge, rotation precise gentle movements are the basic principles of suturing.

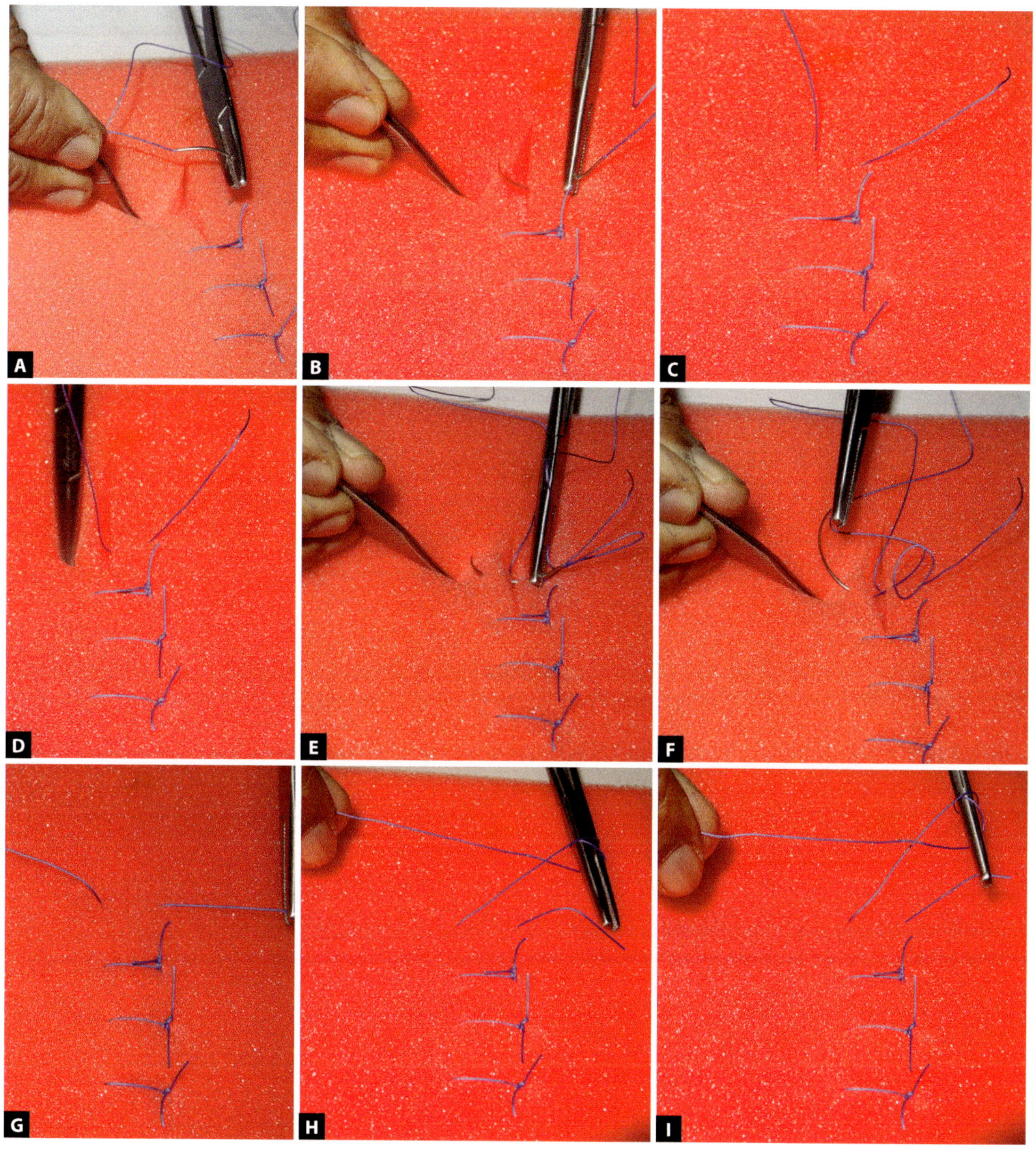

**Figs. 12A to I**

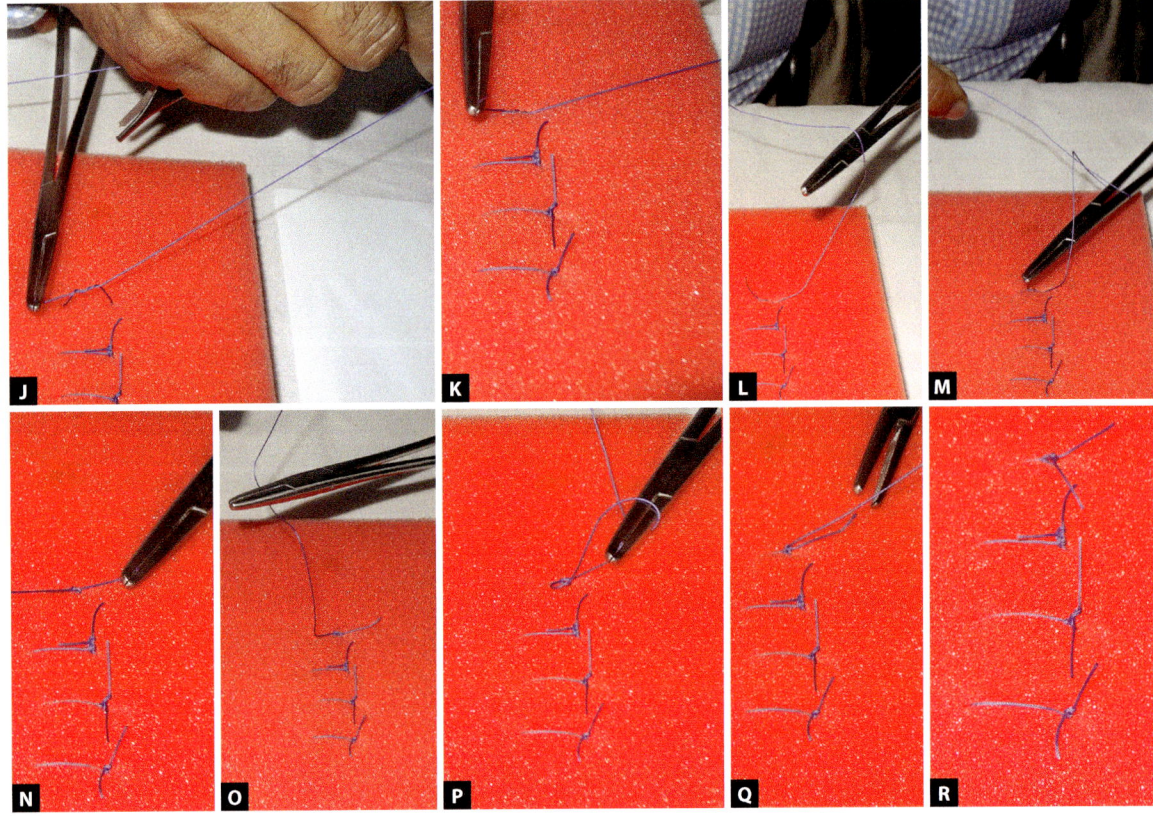

**Figs. 12J to R**

**Figs. 12A to R:** Simple interrupted suture placement technique—step by step.

absorbable sutures. Rapid healing, least irritation is achieved by smaller-sized, monofilament, and inert suture material. In bowel, absorbable suture material used—3-0 is ideal; often 2-0 is also used. Silk is also used in many centers. Interrupted sutures are better especially in esophagus, colorectum, and contaminated field. Continuous sutures are used in stomach, jejunum. Single layer is well accepted; it gives wider lumen; and maintains blood supply. Double layer using silk/linen for outer seromuscular; full thickness Connell/Gambee sutures for inner layer using absorbable sutures such as 3-0 vicryl is also equally good. It is time consuming and may lessen the luminal diameter. But it is more secure. In biliary tree and urinary system, rapidly absorbable sutures such as 3-0 vicryl are used. Patient age, nutrition, immunosuppression, malignancy, sepsis, and acute nature—are other factors which decide the type of suture material used.

*Jenkin's rule:* Suture length to wound length ratio should be at least 4 : 1 often may be even 6:1 as skin and soft tissues lengthen significantly under strain; to accommodate this lengthening, lengthier suture material is needed.

*Removal of the suture:* Different parts of the body heal at different time and different speed. So nonabsorbable skin stitches are

### PRINCIPLES OF SUTURING

- The needle should be grasped at approximately 1/3rd distance from the eye and 2/3rd from point.
- The needle should pierce the tissue perpendicular to its surface.
- The needle should be placed equidistant (2–3 mm) from the incision line.
- The depth of penetration should be equal on both sides of incision line.
- The needle always should pass from movable tissue to the fixed tissue; from thinner tissue to the thicker tissue. In deeper tissues from depth towards superficial.
- Needle should be passed along its curve.
- The tissue should never be closed under tension.
- The bite should be equal on both sides of the wound margin and the point of the entry of the needle should be closer to the wound edge than its point of exit on the deep surface to create flask-shaped suture.
- Should not leave dead space while suturing.
- Each suture must be placed 3–4 mm apart from the incision line.
- Tie the suture to approximate; not to blanch or strangulate.
- Knot must not lie on incision line.
- The distance between one suture to another should be about 3–4 mm apart to prevent strangulation of the tissue and to allow escape of the serum or inflammatory exudate to get more strength of the wound.
- Sutures should be placed at a greater depth than distance from the incision to evert wound margins.
- Deep wounds should be closed in layers.
- Needle tip should not be retrieved by instruments; needle should be held proximal to the tip while retrieving.
- Adequate tissue bite should be taken to prevent tearing.
- Sutures should have correct tension while tying knot with provision for slight edema that occur postoperatively, more tension in sutures cause ischemia of the edges leading into tearing of the tissues.
- Overlapping of suture edge should be avoided.
- Dog ear formation should be avoided; this is done by undermining the extra tissue and incision is extended over this undermined tissue with 30° angulation to original wound and sutured as angle which corrects the dog ear.
- Holding the suture material using needle holder unnecessarily should be avoided. It is held only during knotting process.

## REMEMBER ABOUT SUTURING

- Width of the bite of suture on each side of the wound edge should be equal—*coarse* adjustment.
- Gap between the sutures should be equal. It may be 1 cm gap in skin; 3–5 mm gap in bowel; 1–2 mm gap in vessel.
- Slight eversion of the wound edge causes proper apposition. Scar will be cosmetically acceptable.
- Deeper bite in the tissue by the needle should be wider than superficial to achieve adequate eversion.
- Inversion of edges may cause overlapping, delayed healing, delayed wound gap and poor scarring.
- Knot should be on one side of the bites on the wound bite point; and this knot should be on the stronger side of the wound edges. This is achieved by fine adjustment prior to placing the first throw of the knot.
- Bites should be adequate and deep enough; superficial unequal bites will cause improper apposition.
- Thumb can be used to push the skin against the needle bite from opposite side.
- Suturing is done from more mobile edge of the wound toward relatively immobile side.
- Flap of the tissue/skin when sutured, knot should be on the opposite side of the edge of the flap.
- Vertical mattress sutures give a good eversion.
- Improper alignment of the wound edges in a curved or lengthy wounds can be prevented by placing the key sutures at salient points which are identified by holding the edges taut using skin hooks or marking corresponding points on each edge to have proper alignment and to prevent distortion.
- Wound tension should be distributed equally.
- Optimum tension at suture line will not cause blanching of the skin and will only leave thin/least suture mark whereas more tension with abnormally tight suture will blanch the skin causing obvious suture mark.
- Apposition, not strangulation of the tissues should be done. Optimum tension and adequate number of stitches should be used. Excessive stitches should be avoided.
- Matching and alignment of wound edges are important. Dog ear should be avoided. In lengthy wound, first suture is placed centrally; next one is between end of the wound and the first suture; this will allow proper apposition and avoids dog ear formation.
- Curve of the needle should be followed; levering causes damage.
- Least tissue trauma, atraumatic handling, optimum precision are the need.
- Suturing and knotting is an art; a craft; and is a fine work.
- First bite should be slow, precise, careful and best bite; should not be rapid, clumsy bite and one should avoid repetition.
- Matching landmarks on either side of the wound should be identified properly.
- Suturing is easier with multifilament suture material such as silk than monofilament suture material. Silk has got best handling ability, knot holding property, and least memory. Suture insertion and passage through tissues is easier with silk.
- Tissues should be handled gently; heavy retraction of the tissues should be avoided.
- Proper selection of sutures and needles is important.
- Layers should be approximated properly but as tension free (layer by layer).
- Dead space should be obliterated.
- Skin and tough structures such as periosteum needs cutting needles; atraumatic eyeless needle with sutures are ideal.
- Interrupted sutures are better whenever there is edema, infection/inflammation or in secondary suturing. Nonabsorbable monofilament sutures are advisable here.
- Subcuticular or absorbable sutures are used in clean wounds.

*Note:* After act of suturing, needle should be returned to scrub nurse with needle holder.

removed at different periods in different places—face: 5 days; over joints: 14 days; trunk: 10 days; scalp: 7–10 days; and secondary sutured stitches: 14 days.

### USE OF LIGATURE

Ligation of bleeding vessel is essential in many places. Small vessel is cauterized after holding with hemostat. Wider vessel should be ligated. Polyglycolic acid 2-0 or 3-0 can be used. Silk also can be used as it holds well with good strength. Once surgeon places the first knot (throw), assistant *gently* releases the hemostat and removes it. Hemostat should not be released suddenly.

*Mounted tie* is used for small or medium vein ligation. Here two ligatures are placed with 0.5 or 1 cm gap around the vein using two hemostats and tied securely. Vein in-between is cut safely **(Fig. 13)**. If it is artery two ligatures are placed proximally and one ligature distally before cutting in-between. Larger vein ligation also needs double ligation proximally.

Ligating the larger vessel such as left gastric artery, branches of mesenteric vessel and superior thyroid artery needs additional care as slippage in reality is a definitive risk. In such occasions, ideal method could be to dissect the vessel from adjacent tissue and fat for 1.5 cm (*skeletonization of the vessel*) length and ligating it. Ligation of such vessel needs special care. Initially, vessel is cross-clamped using *Mixter/Miegster* clamp **(Fig. 14)**. Using long hemostat lengthy ligature (silk or polyglycolic acid) is passed around the Mixter clamp and tied using hand knot. One more ligature is placed again 2 mm proximal to earlier ligature. Stump of the vessel should be around >0.5 mm up to 10 mm beyond the distal ligature.

Often in resection of the tissue such as gastrectomy, mastectomy, colectomy, intestinal resection, main vessel (gastric artery/gastroepiploic artery/mesenteric

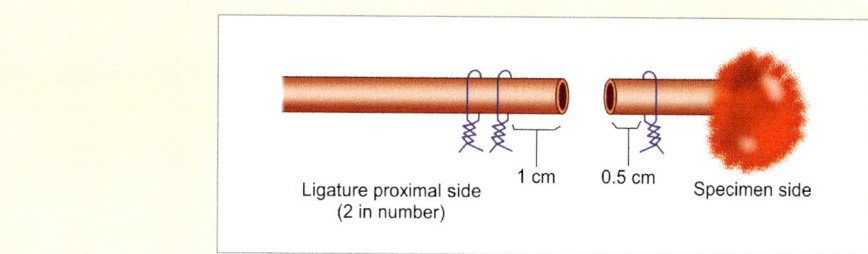

**Fig. 13:** Vessel is cut between knots with adequate gap in-between to prevent knot slippage. Ideally proximal two ligations and distal one ligation are needed.

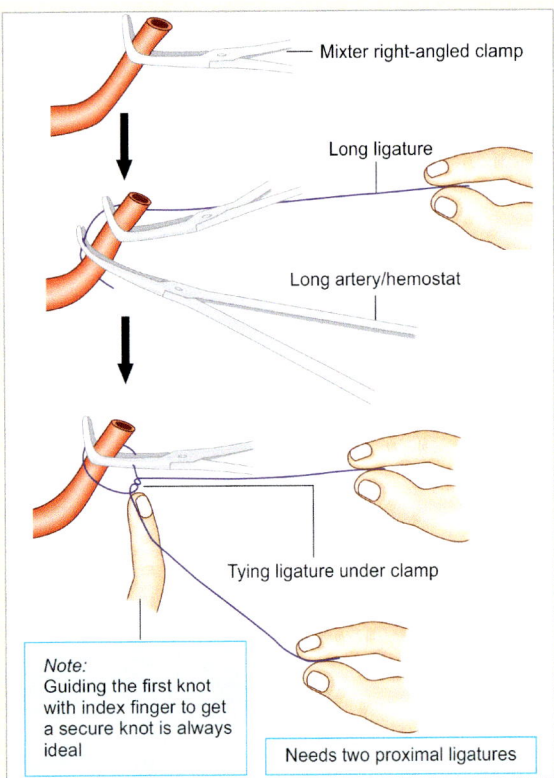

**Fig. 14:** In the depth, vessel should be dissected first properly. Mixter/Miegster clamp is applied. Ligature is passed underneath using long hemostat. Ligature is placed by firm knot which is directed using index finger.

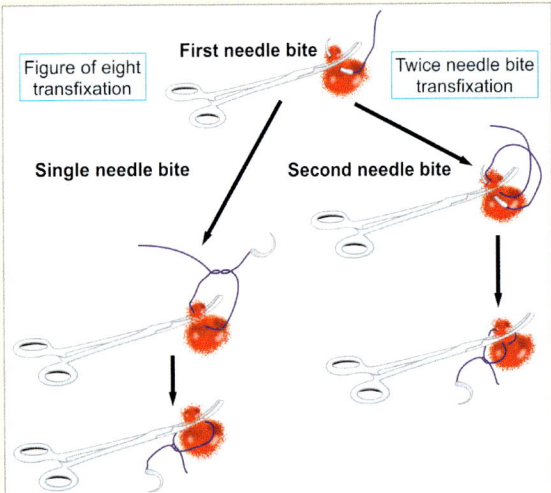

**Fig. 15:** Transfixation suture. By two methods, it is done. Single bite, figure of eight suture or double bite transfixation is used. Both hold knots in place with minimal chance for slippage.

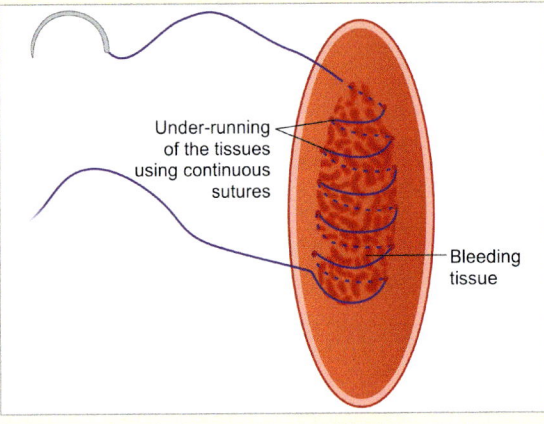

**Fig. 16:** Under-running of tissues.

vessel branch) is isolated and dissected for about 2 cm length and ligature is passed using Mixter clamp as a feeding ligature and tied. Proximal two ligatures are placed at 2 mm apart. Distal ligature is placed away at 1.5 cm gap. Vessel is cut using curved scissor or with No. 15 blade (part behind the vessel should be guarded by placing flat surface of the dissecting forceps or any other instrument) leaving 1 cm vessel proximally and 0.5 cm vessel distally. Two firm proper proximal ligatures are sufficient even though many surgeons have got the habit of placing three or more proximal ligatures. Only one proximal ligature is technically sufficient but is not advisable; so two proximal ligatures are probably ideal.

## TRANSFIXATION LIGATURE

Transfixation prevents the slippage of the suture. It is used in big vessel ligation or when oozing tissues are held and ligated. Gastric vessels, mesenteric branches, in obese patients where ligature may not hold, in vessels in the depth—are the indications. It is better to use transfixation suture whenever surgeon feels that just ligature may not be sufficient to secure.

Needle with the suture is passed underneath the hemostat over middle of the grasped tissue, first knot encircles half of the tissue on one side; suture is looped around on the opposite side of the grasped tissue and knot is placed. Once such *figure of eight stitch* is complete, then only hemostat is released by the assistant. Further knots are placed over it. Still safety of the ligature can be achieved by passing the needle *second time* underneath the tissue again before knotting **(Fig. 15)**.

## UNDER-RUNNING OF THE TISSUE

It is not possible to catch the area and control the bleeding, if bleeding point is not identified and is not pointed. Any blind struggle to hold the area with hemostat will aggravate the bleeding without achieving anything. In such occasion, it is wiser to place continuous locking sutures in tissue bed where bleeding occurs using 3-0 polyglycolic acid/silk/polypropylene sutures. Repeated mopping and suction of the area is essential. However, surgeon should take care and be aware of presence of some major vessels and vital structures in that deeper plane. Depth control in these sutures is also important. Usually, bleeding stops by placing few locking sutures. Locked loops should be held by the surgeon himself so that tearing through the tissues by the suture material is avoided and gentle traction to lift the tissue to facilitate further bites is achieved **(Fig. 16)**.

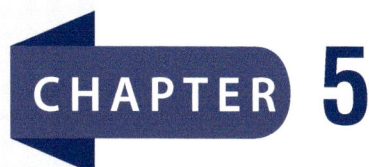

# CHAPTER 5

# Surgical Knot Tying

> "Wherever the art of medicine is loved, there is also a love of humanity."
> –Hippocrates

## INTRODUCTION

A *knot* connects two ends strongly so as to hold them without any chance of slippage. *Knots* are classified as decorative knot and utility knot. *Decorative knots* are ornamental and are of least surgical importance. *Utility knots* are strong, reliable, and secure. Knots used in surgical practice are utility knots. Hitches, bends, stopper knots, loop, and running knots are different knots. Hitch knots are used to tie around an object which may be crossing knots (clove hitch knot) or rolling knots. Bend knot is used to join two ends. A loop is a multistrand bend knot. Knots have strength/efficiency, security, and capsizing, slipping, and sliding properties.

*Components of knot are:* Bight (loop between ends), bitter end (end which is tied off), loop (open or closed), elbow, turn (turn may be single turn/round turn/two-round turn), working end, and working part.

There are so many knots that are used for various purposes: Domestic, professional, various work places, and surgical fields. The knot is named according to its use.

*Different stopper knots are:* Overhand/half-knot, multiple overhand knot, figure-of-eight knot, and heaving line knot.

Knots are tied either using instrument (instrument tie) or using hands. Hand ties need lengthy sutures when compared to instrument tie. Knotting for surface sutures is usually done using instrument tie. Knotting requires proper wrist and elbow movements, ergonomics, proper knot holding, and adequate throws (minimum three; in certain monofilament sutures such as polypropylene, it is five). The knot should maintain optimum strength at the wound apposition site, but it should not strangulate the tissue edge.

*Note:*
- Secure knotting is the most difficult part in tissue approximation whether in open or laparoscopic method.
- That is why so many different methods of knotting techniques have evolved for different tissues, and it is rather difficult to remember all. Surgeon should be well versed with required essential methods of knotting in day-to-day surgical practice but important to remember is it should be perfect.

## PRINCIPLES

The knot must be simple, firmly tied, and should not slip. Knots must be as small as possible and ends should be cut as short as possible in the tissues. Skin sutures which are to be removed should be kept around 0.5–1 cm in length so that removal becomes easier since keeping too long sutures will abut into adjacent knots causing problem.

When two ends are being tied together, they must be of the same material and same caliber. The *"sheet bend"* knot **(Fig. 1)** is the only knot which is safer to tie in two dissimilar materials.

In tying the knot, one should avoid friction between strands to avoid weakening of the suture and avoid damage to the suture while tying the knot.

Excessive tension while tying the knot will lead to suture breakage or tissue damage. Strength should be optimum, neither too tight nor too loose. Beginners tend to put too tight knots. Too tight sutures may cause tissue strangulation.

After tying the first loop, tension should be maintained on the strand to avoid loosening of knot. The final throw should be as nearly horizontal as possible. The surgeon should not hesitate to change stance or position in order to place a secure flat knot. Usually, three knots are sufficient. The first knot is the best knot. In retention sutures or if polypropylene is used as suture material, then a maximum of four/five knots have to be placed. Any additional knot will not help in stability of knot or do not add to the strength of a securely tied square knot.

Often, the first throw/knot can be gently pushed and guided using the index finger **(Fig. 2)**. Squaring the knot is very essential **(Fig. 3)**.

Sutures should have correct tension while tying the knot for provision of postoperative slight edema; more tensioned sutures can cause ischemia of the edges and tearing of the tissues, may leave suture mark, and the edges may get overlapped. While putting knots, *over and under wrapping sequence* should never be violated.

In continuous sutures, *starter and terminal knots* are important as these two knots hold and give strength to the wound. The starter knot is placed by classical reef square knot; the terminal knot is placed using an instrument needle holder by looping into the end of the closed loop of the last bite. Aberdeen knot is a terminal knot.

The suture material part adjacent to the swage of the needle is called *rear end*; it continues as *leading part of the suture material*; the end of the suture material is called *trailing end of the suture* which stays toward the side of the beginning on the needle bite to place the knot **(Figs. 4A and B)**.

*While knotting*, forceps should be held reverse in the palm of the surgeon's hand (left hand in a right-hand surgeon) and needle and leading part of the suture material should be held loose in the palm of the same hand in front of the forceps **(Figs. 5A to C)**.

*Sutured knot has got three components:* (1) Loop created by knot, (2) knot itself

### PRINCIPLES OF KNOT TYING
- Simplest knot that prevents slippage should be used.
- Tying the knot as small as possible and cutting the ends of the suture as short as reasonable minimize foreign body reaction.
- One should avoid friction or sawing.
- One should avoid damage to suture material.
- Excessive tension should be avoided.
- Tying sutures too tightly strangulates the tissue.
- Traction should be maintained at one end of the suture after the first loop is thrown to avoid loosening of the knot.
- Final throw should be placed as horizontally as possible to keep knot flat.
- Limiting extra throws to the knot is important as they do not add strength to a properly tied knot.
- Knot should be on one side of the sutured wound; it should not be on the wound line.

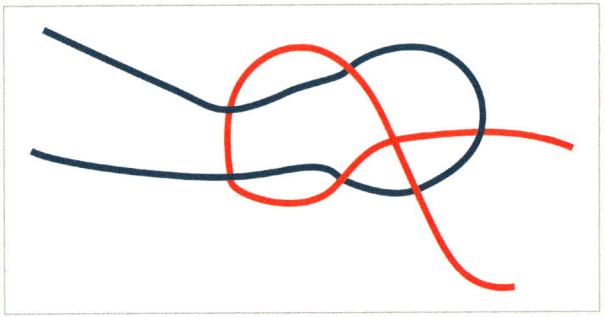

**Fig. 1:** Sheet bend knot.

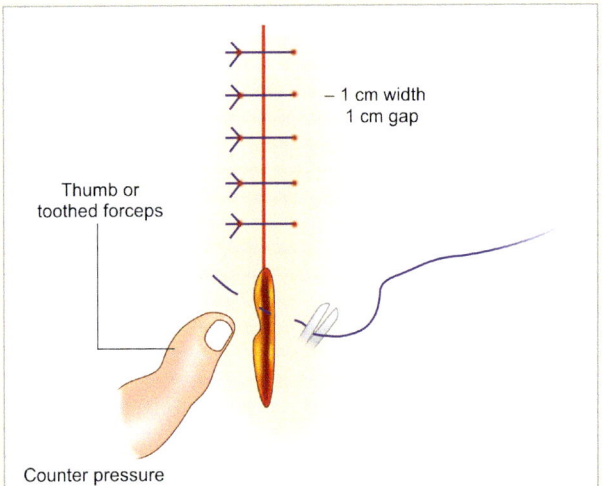

**Fig. 2:** First throw/knot should be gently pushed and guided using the index finger.

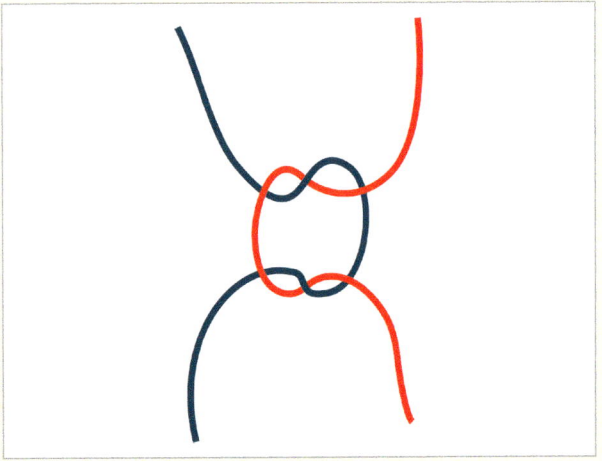

**Fig. 3:** Squaring the knot is very essential.

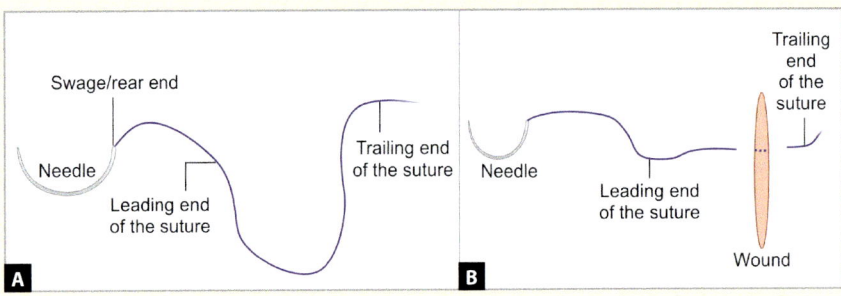

**Figs. 4A and B:** *Parts of the suture material:* Rear end, leading part, and trailing end of the suture material.

which is composed of a number of tight throws, and (3) ears which are the cut ends of the suture **(Fig. 6)**.

## STAGES OF KNOT TYING

There are three stages while tying the knot: (1) *Configuration* is tying the knot, (2) *shaping the knot* is working/drawing the knot, and (3) *securing the knot* is snuggling or locking the knot.

## DIFFERENT TYPES OF KNOTS

- *Reef (square) knot:* It is done with squaring and is ideal and commonly used knot. The first two throws are pulled in opposite directions to square the knot. Correct squaring is essential, otherwise the knot gets spoiled and loosened **(Figs. 7A and B)**.
- *Granny knot:* Here first two throws are pulled in the same direction with the second loop being taken from the same side. It is mainly used when two throws are placed and cinched across down toward the tissue to tighten the lock to create granny knot. It is not as secure as square knot; it has tendency to slip **(Fig. 8)**.
- *Surgeon's knot* with one extra loop in the first knot with squaring. It prevents loosening and slipping of the knot and maintains strength and tension required with the tissue and so becomes a more secure knot **(Fig. 9)**.
- *Modified Fisherman's knot:* First knot has got three loops/throws with surgeon's knot with squaring; second knot is squared single loop; third knot is squared double throw surgeon's knot.
- *Triple modified reef knot:* It is the reef with three knots instead of two. It is actually the commonly used knot **(Figs. 10 and 11)**.
- *Self-locking suture knot:* It is used as end knot usually used while closing deeper tissue such as rectus sheath or aponeurosis in the abdominal wall. It gives adequate strength and does not slip and used while finishing the continuous suture **(Fig. 12)**.

## DIFFERENT KNOT TYING TECHNIQUES

Hand knots and instrument knots are used. In different situations, different types of knots are used. In the depth, hand knots may be preferred as knots can be quickly done and slid toward the depth using index finger. Two-hands technique, single-hand technique, and Aberdeen method are used.

### Hand Knot Tying

Two-hands and single-hand techniques are used. Two-hands technique is ideal.

Surgical Knot Tying

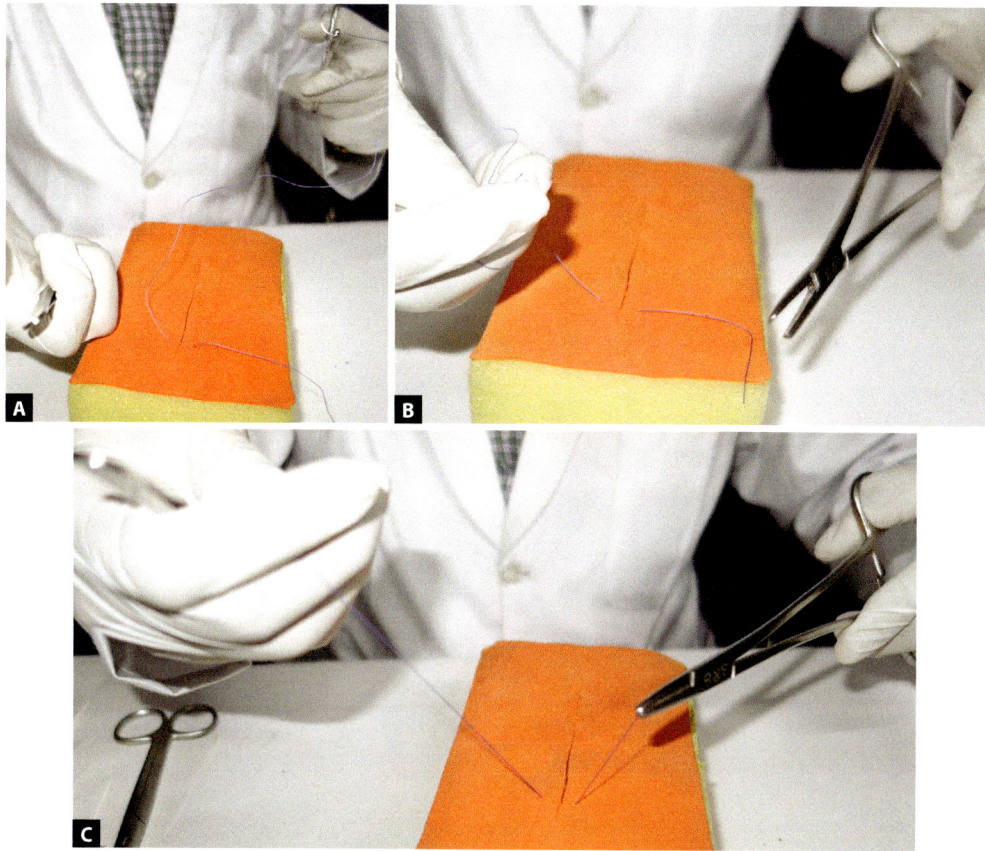

**Figs. 5A to C:** Holding the forceps and needle during knotting.

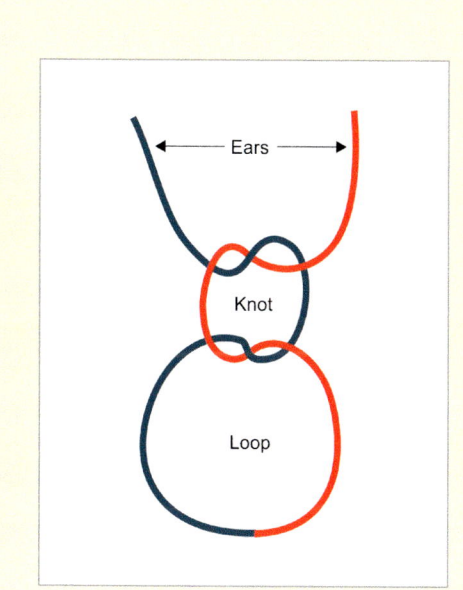

**Fig. 6:** *Components of a knot:* (1) Loop, (2) Knot, and (3) Ears.

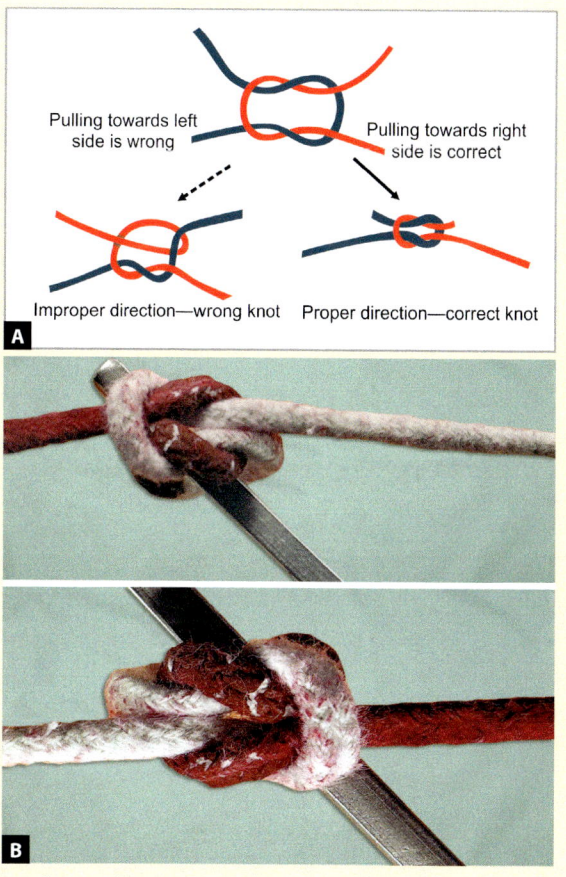

**Figs. 7A and B:** Reef knot. First two throws are pulled in opposite directions to square the loop and tightened to achieve the locking. Third throw is also placed as a support.

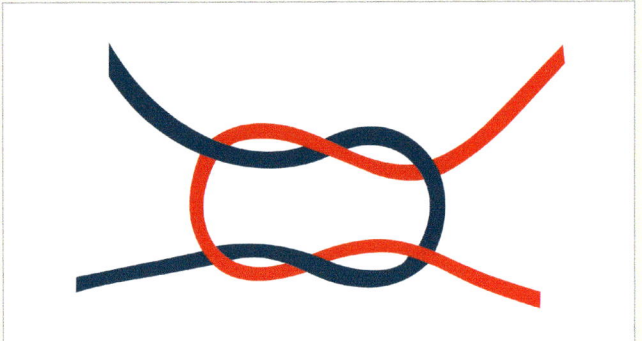

**Fig. 8:** Granny knot. It is not commonly used.

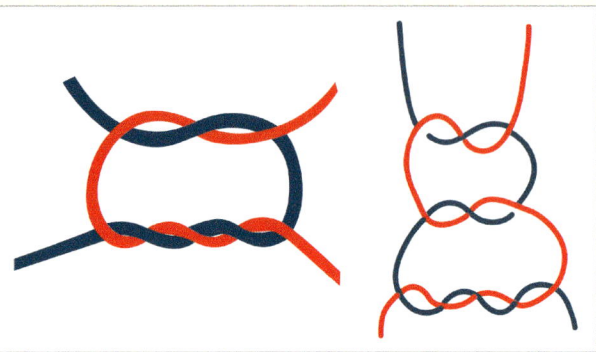

**Fig. 9:** Typical surgeon's knot is taking two loops/throws in first knot with squaring. It holds well without slippage.

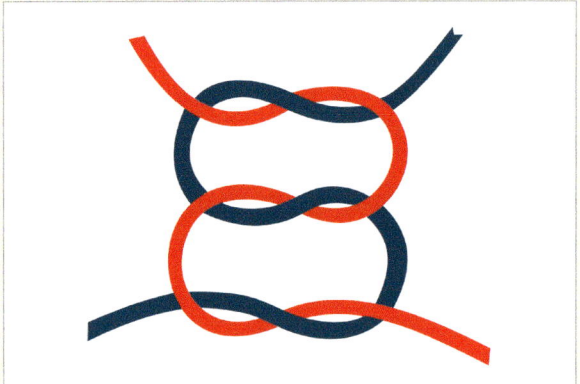

**Fig. 10:** Reef with three knots is used here which is more secure.

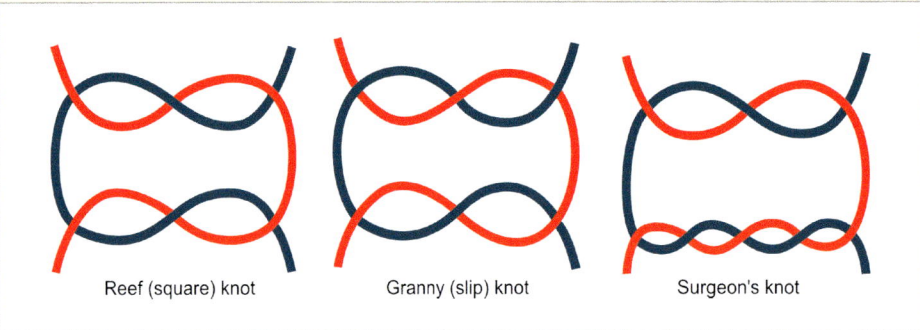

**Fig. 11:** Different types of knots used commonly in surgery—comparison.

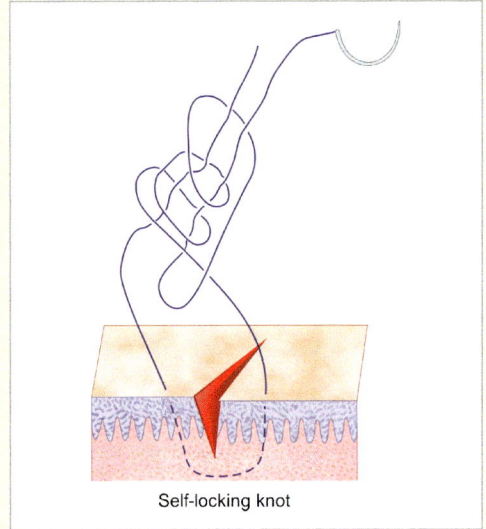

**Fig. 12:** Self-locking suture knot. It is used as end knot usually used while closing deeper tissue such as rectus sheath or aponeurosis in the abdominal wall. Here it is shown in the skin as illustration.

# Surgical Knot Tying

## Two-hands Technique

Two-hands technique is easier hand knot (after practice) **(Figs. 13A to Q)**. With the left hand between thumb and index finger, one end of the thread is held (held proximal to the pulp of these two fingers) with loop coming in front from below; other end of the thread holding in right hand is passed across index finger of left hand coming from behind up and forward close to the other end of the thread in left hand; apposed pulps of the thumb and index finger is looped around it and left hand thread tip is passed between these two finger pulps to achieve the knot. Further knots are repeated similarly. Surgical knots can also be placed. Knots can be placed in similar way by single-hand technique.

## Single-hand Technique

Single-hand technique is done using left hand index finger and/or index and middle fingers. Thread is held similarly but between left thumb and left middle finger, looping is done using left index finger. This method is used whenever the thread is small or there is less space in the area. It is little cumbersome to do when compared to two-hands technique **(Figs. 14A to K)**. It is done using left hand in right-hander; end of the thread/suture material is held between thumb and index finger of left hand; this part of the thread will pass behind the little finger of left hand, encircling it, and coming forward toward between thumb and index finger. Opposite end of the thread which is held in right hand is looped in front across middle finger; middle finger is stretched and holding this right hand loop will be flexed at the distal interphalangeal joint and looped around the left hand thread end to create first knot which is held between apposed middle and ring fingers. These two fingers with the thread are pulled toward left to release the knot; knot is squared by directing the left hand toward the opposite

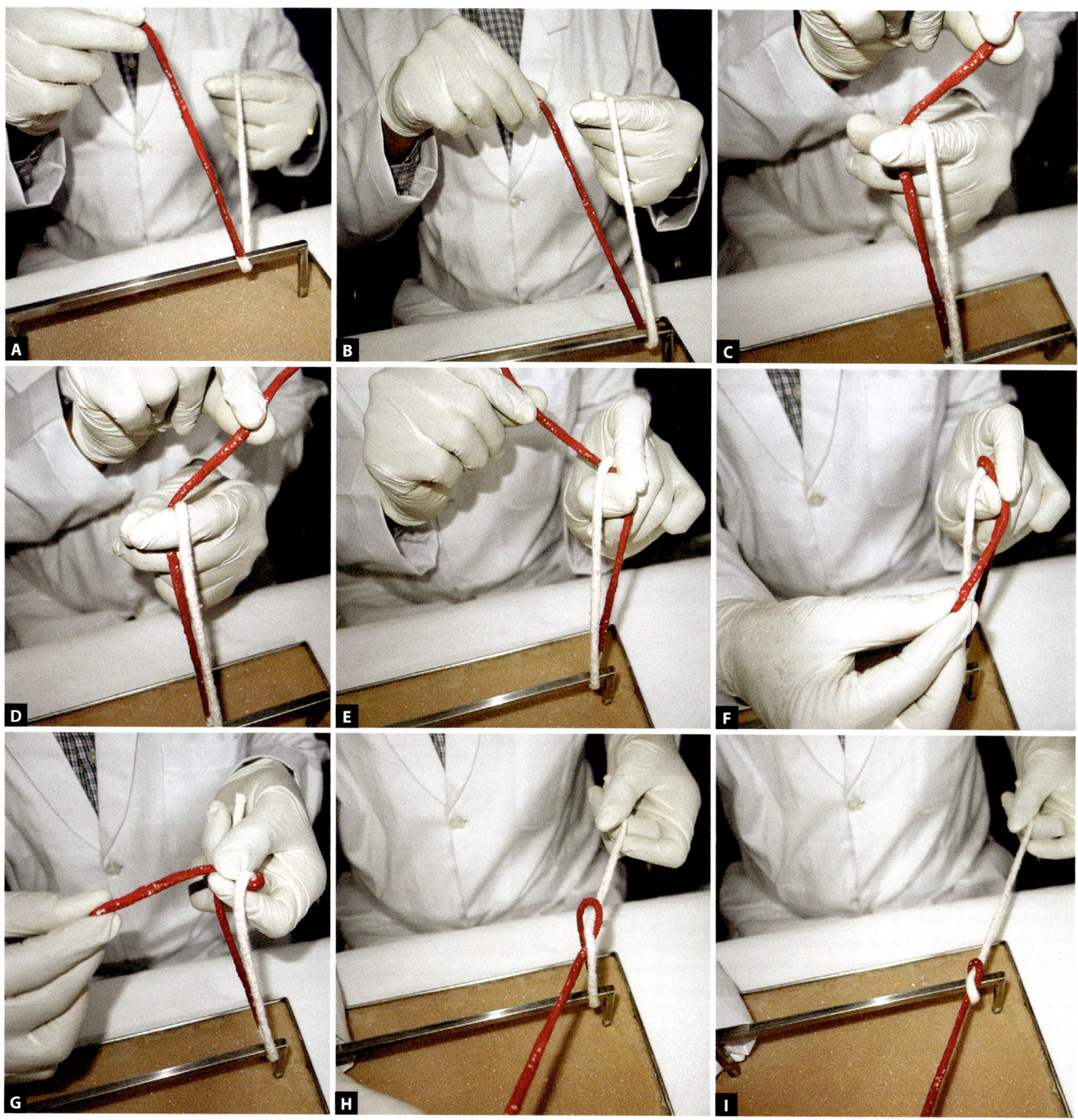

**Figs. 13A to I**

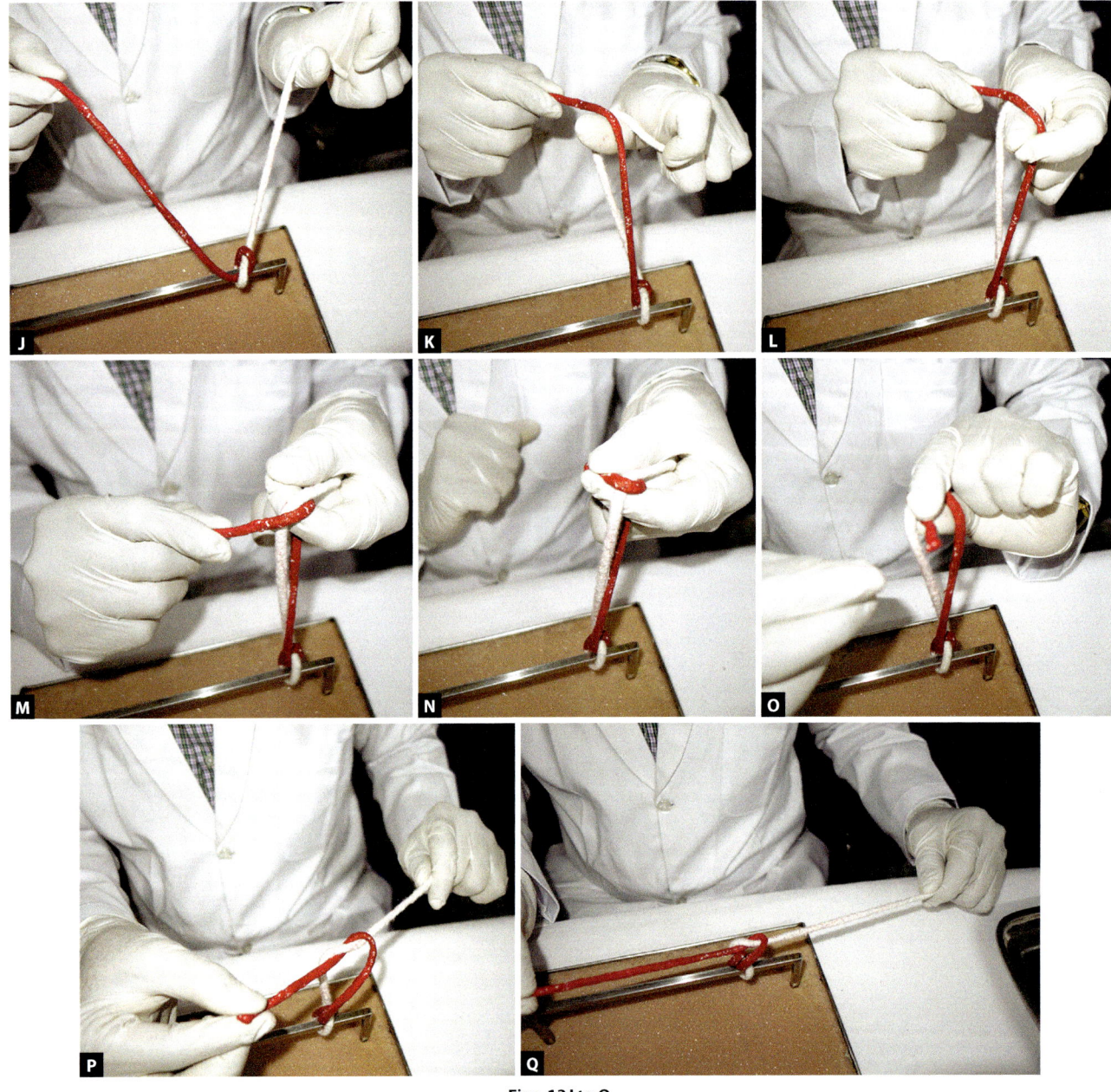

**Figs. 13J to Q**

**Figs. 13A to Q:** Hand knotting using two-hands technique (Two-hand square knot).

side; knot is tightened by gentle push using pulp of left index finger. Further two knots are also placed similarly.

### Aberdeen Hand Knot

*Aberdeen hand knot* is also used to end the continuous suture **(Figs. 15A to M)**. It is *"chain stitch knot,"* which is a self-locking knot used in continuous suture pattern. It is used as end knot. End (last loop of continuous suture) loop is held open with one hand; leading end of the suture (one which is on needle end) is looped and passed through the loop from the last bite which is already held; such similar loops are passed through the loop on loop for several times. Usually after five to six loops, leading end of the suture material with its needle is passed through the last final loop and pulled tight to finish the Aberdeen knot. The Aberdeen knot became so named when Sir James Learmonth (Professor of Surgery at *Aberdeen University* from 1932 to 1938) noted that it used less thread than the contemporary surgeon's knot. Actually, it is pulling free leading end of the suture through the loop thus creating a new loop when it is looped and such loop throws are repeated ideally for six times and at the end, needle with leading suture end is passed through the final loop and locked with a pull to complete the knot. *Laparoscopic Aberdeen knot* is also used.

### Instrument Knot Tying

This is the basic essentiality for surgery. There are different types of knot tying methods depending on loops taken, squaring, throws, etc. The needle holder should be held parallel to the tissue/surface. It is held with one hand (dominant hand); long limb side (leading end) of the suture is held with other hand (nondominant hand) usually at around 10 cm from the swaged end of the needle; needle is allowed to hang down freely so that needle injury is avoided. The instrument (needle holder) is looped/wrapped (throws) around the suture (leading side), usually twice for a surgical knot [first (half) knot ideally should be *surgical knot* when tissues are in tension, which means two loops are taken]; the needle driver/holder is moved toward the trailing end of the suture to grasp it near its end (without allowing

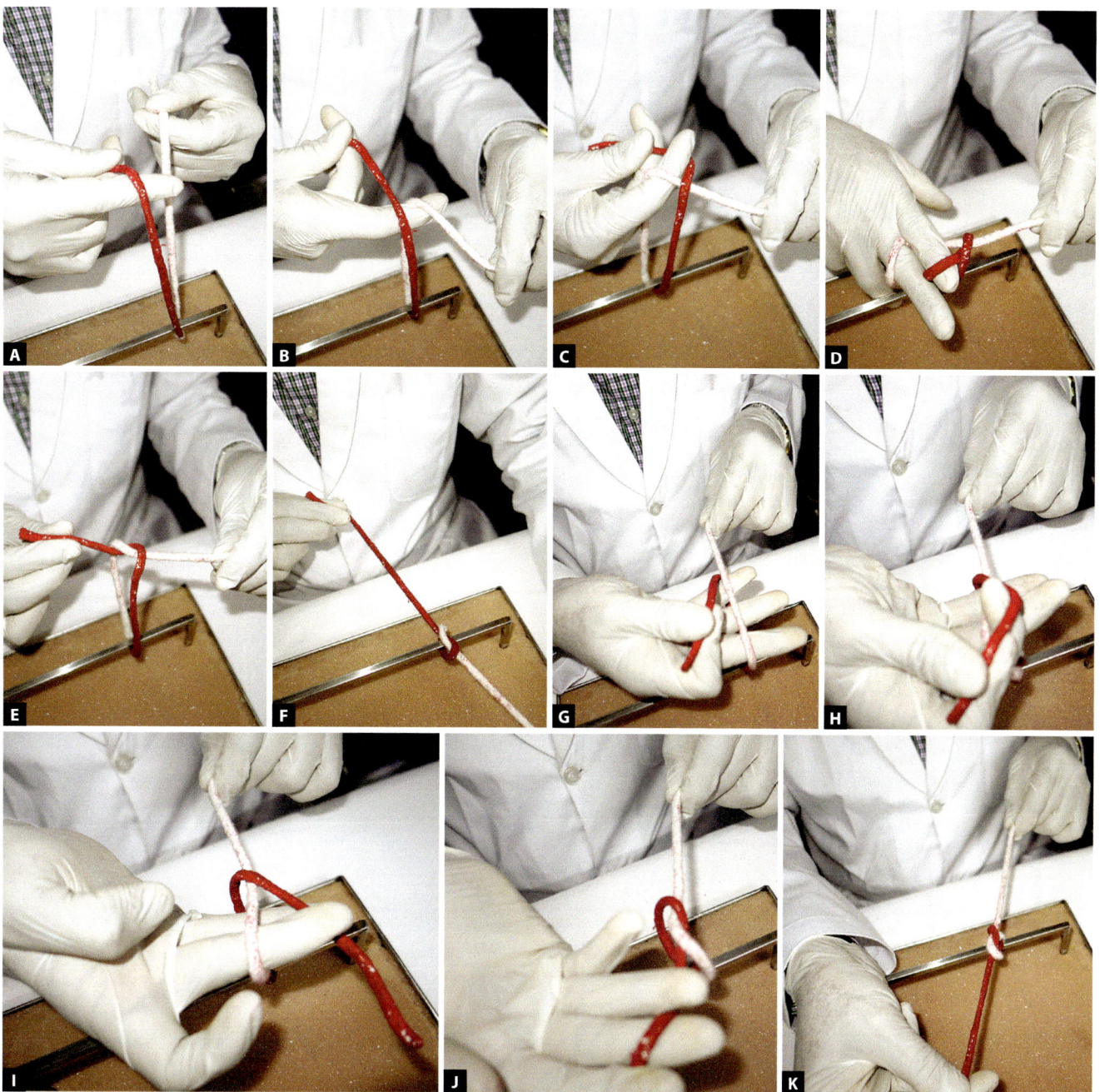

**Figs. 14A to K:** Making knot with single-hand technique. Surgeon should learn this technique as it is used when suture ends are short.

any movement of the wrapped looped leading end). The instrument is crossed to opposite side perpendicular to the wound edge to square the knot and gently knot is tightened; tightening of the knot should be adequate enough which means neither too tight to strangulate the tissue nor too loose to create a gap. This first knot (half knot) is the *essential knot* in knotting; gentle traction should be held to the leading strand (leading end) to avoid loosening of the first knot; two ends of the suture should be pulled in opposite directions with equal gentle traction. The second knot is taken as a single loop which is usually taken from behind the suture material (opposite direction and squared in opposite direction in reef knotting) and is tightened **(Figs. 16A to J)**; third knot is again single loop (or often double loop like surgeon's knot) **(Figs. 17A to J)** taken from front of the suture material (alike first knot single or double loop) and is tightened. One has to remember that usually three firm proper knots are sufficient. It is always considered that even though first (half) knot is the holding knot, total two (half) knots (only one additional knot) are *insufficient* and *so three (half) knots are essential*. Each throw is considered as half knot; so, to complete a knot, minimum two throws are required; adding one more throw creates three throws which are ideally needed. If first and second throws of the knot are taken from same side without squaring it becomes granny knot (in reef knot 1st and 2nd throws are taken from opposite sides **(Figs. 18A to G)**.

Only suture material like polypropylene which has highest *memory* (recoiling tendency and so poor knot holding ability), four to five knots are placed. Any further additional knots will not help in strengthening the knot further; so it is a waste of energy by the surgeon and unnecessary creating bunch in the knot. After placing the first knot, it is always better to fix the knot with surgeon's index finger to confirm the adequacy of tightness of the knot.

*Instrumental knotting is* more precise than hand knotting; as it creates optimum regulated tension at the suture line; and knot guidance and placement is better with instrument.

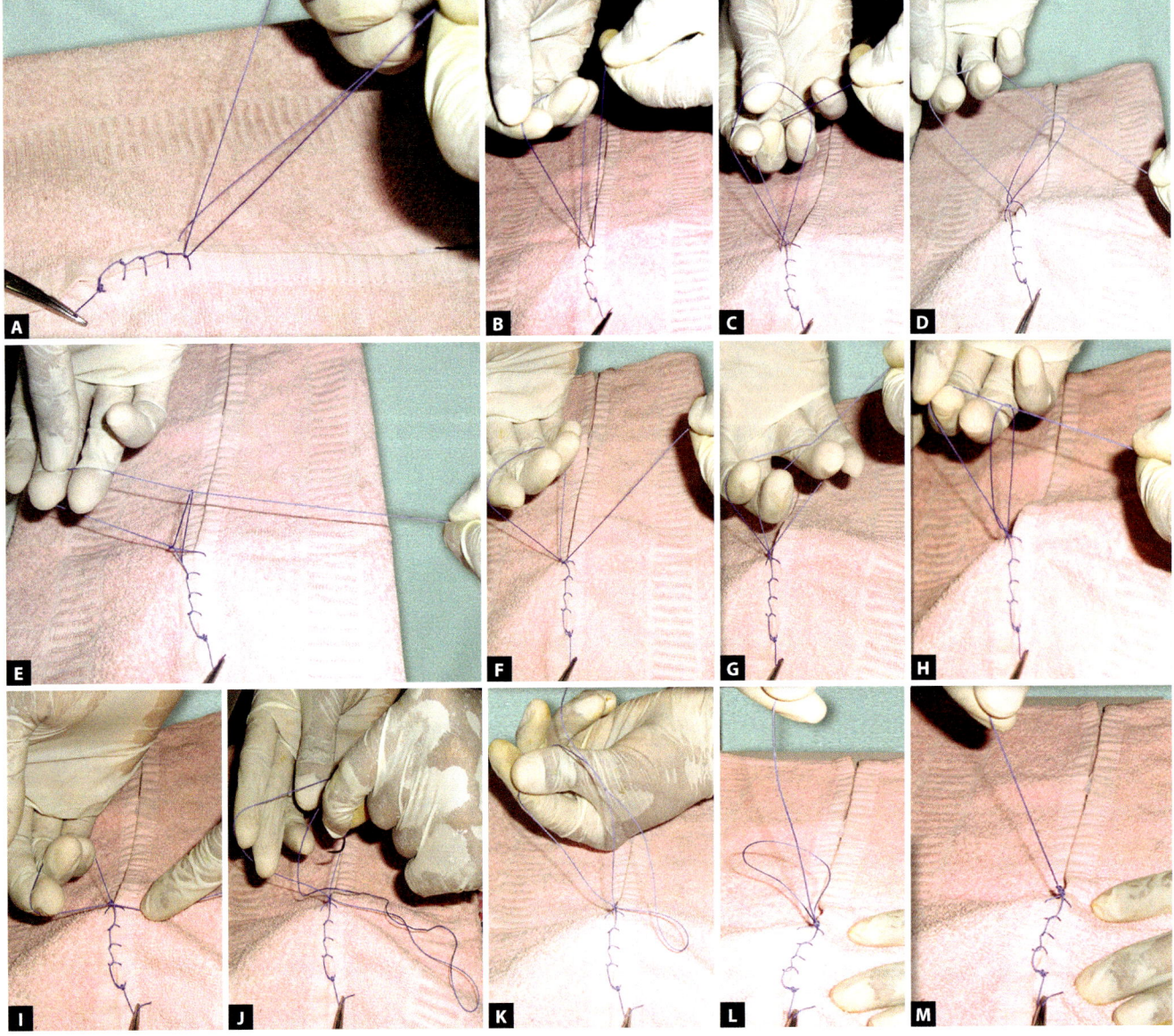

**Figs. 15A to M:** Aberdeen knotting (Aberdeen University in Scotland).

### REMEMBER

- Optimum grip, optimum control, and optimum precision are essential.
- Hold the suture with needle holder only during knotting (not in other time).
- Knot must be as small as possible.
- In skin after knotting ends of interrupted sutures are cut neither too short nor too long; usually 1 cm of length which is equivalent to gap between sutures. In deeper plane, it should be kept short.
- One should avoid friction between strands while knotting. This can be minimized by holding sutures loosely, not tightly like a string. If so, it will cause sawing effect and reduces the strength of the suture.
- Holding the suture with excessive tension will break the suture and traumatize the tissues. Holding with minimum tension allows free movement of the suture for finer suturing.
- First knot (half knot/first throw) is *the important* knot; after placing first knot, gentle traction to the strand is needed to avoid loosening of the first knot. Two ends of the suture should be pulled in opposite directions with equal gentle traction.
- Knotting is for proper apposition and approximation of the tissues; not for strangulation; so too tight suture should be avoided. Optimum tension should be used. This art comes to a surgeon by repeated practice and experience.
- Surgeon should adjust his stance and position to place the knot properly.
- All knots ideally should be squared for stability by pulling in opposite directions.
- Friable edges of the wound cause poor knot holding and placement.
- After placing the knot, ears/ends of the knot should be 5 mm in surface/skin knots. It is around 2–3 mm in deeper plane; if long ears/ends are left, it may penetrate other adjacent tissues; if very small ends/ears (cutting close to the knot) knot throws may slip.

## DOG-EAR

After excision of a circular lesion while closing the wound, the ends of the wound get elevated like pronouncement called as "dog-ear" **(Fig. 19)**." If this is sutured as it is, it causes a prominence resulting in unsatisfactory cosmetic scar. Such wound is sutured until dog-ear is formed; later dog-ear is excised with lengthening of the wound; suturing continued to create lengthier clean sutured wound which eventually leads into a clean scar.

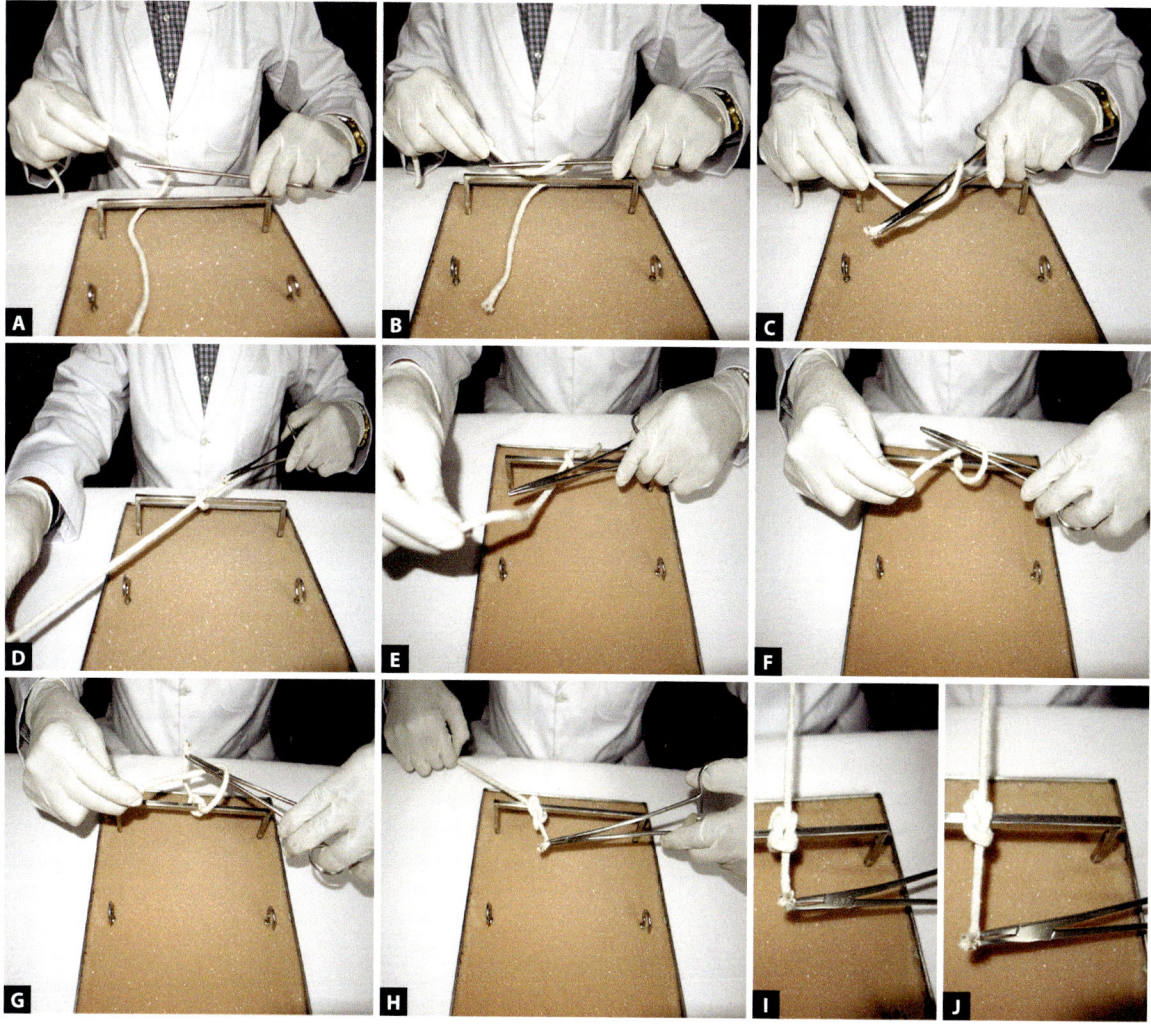

**Figs. 16A to J:** Placing reef knot using needle holder instrument. Knot should be squared for proper secure knot to get.

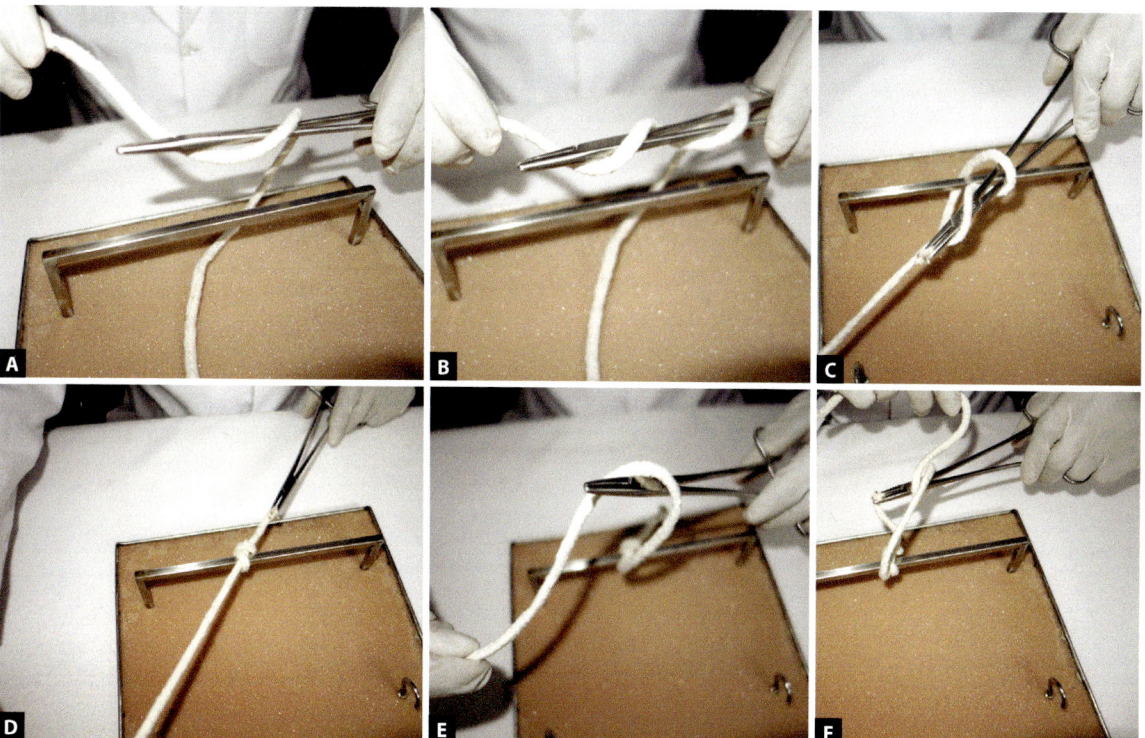

**Figs. 17A to F**

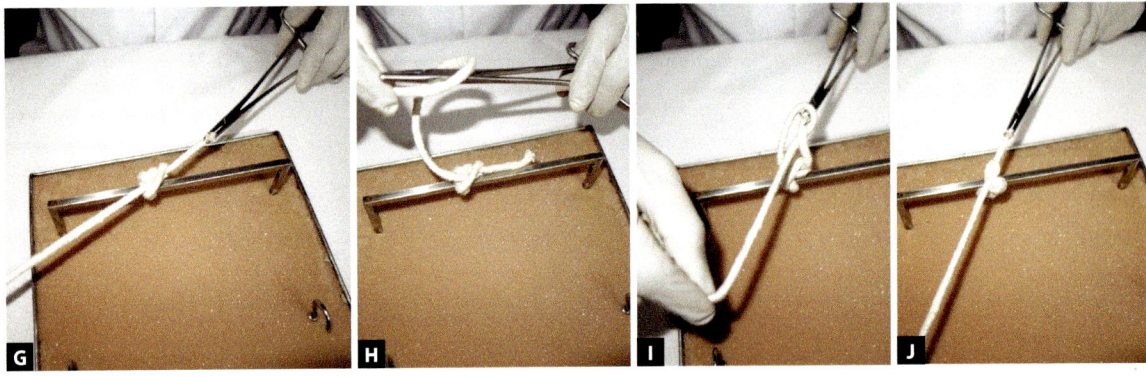

**Figs. 17G to J**

**Figs. 17A to J:** Instrumental placing of surgeon's knot (double throw of first loop with squaring). It is more secure and does not slip; it is ideal in tissues where tension and chances of knot slippage is present.

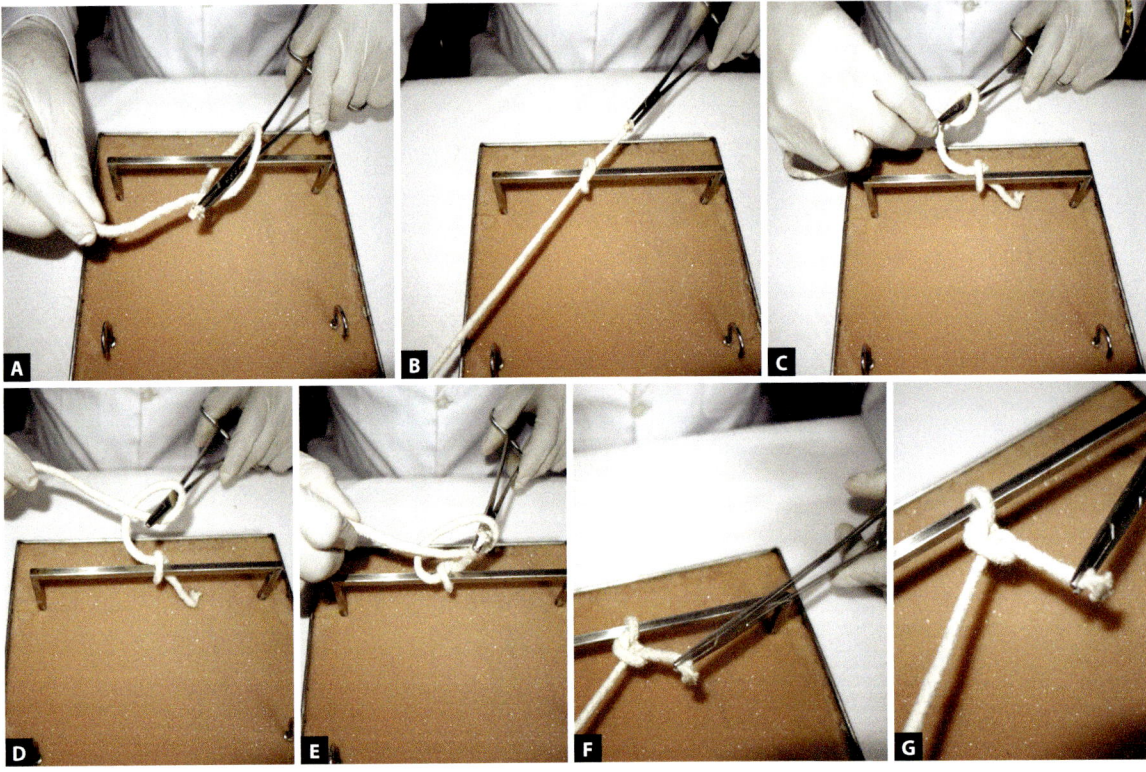

**Figs. 18A to G:** Granny knot using instrument. Here second throw is taken from front same as first throw with pulling in same direction as first throw.

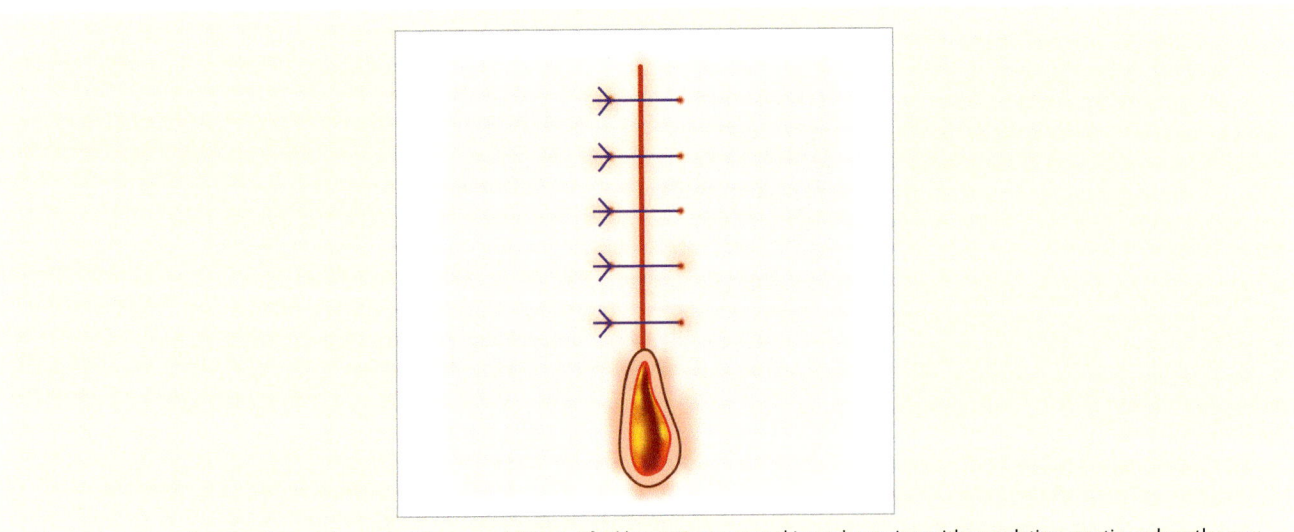

**Fig. 19:** Dog-ear often develops at the end of the wound. It is rectified by cutting excess skin and suturing with angulation creating a lengthy scar.

## SUTURE REMOVAL

Suture cutting scissor is used with sharp tips. Suture is cut on one side deep to the knot; it is pulled using forceps *toward the wound line* so as to prevent entering of the exposed part of the suture to get into the deeper part of suture line during removal and also to prevent wound dehiscence. Cut suture if pulled away, from the wound line, there is higher chances of wound dehiscence. Surgeon should use wrist and finger movements. BP handle with *11 number pointed sharp blade* also can be used. Patient should be always in lying down position. Suture removal is also an art.

If suture is kept long time, problems such as abscess formation, implantation dermoid, stitch mark, and bad scaring can occur. Suture marks are caused by following reasons: Skin sutures left in place >7 days, resulting in epithelialization of suture track; tissue necrosis from sutures that were tied too tightly or became tight due to tissue edema; and use of reactive sutures in the skin.

> *Suture removal is an art. It is done with all aseptic precautions. Suture is cut behind the knot and suture is held at the knot using dissecting forceps or hemostat, pulled towards the wound so that wound dehiscence will not occur and outer part of the suture material is not dragged inside the track during removal to reduce the possible chances of infection along the track.*

# Skin and Soft Tissue Suturing

> *"Progress is man's ability to complicate simplicity".*
> –Thor Heyerdahl, Norwegian Adventurer (1914–2002)

## INTRODUCTION

Even though suturing technique is similar anywhere in the body, suturing of the skin and soft tissues differs in many ways. Skin being a tough structure needs strong cutting needle and a toothed dissecting forceps which is used to hold the skin while suturing. Round bodied needle and toothed forceps or hemostat cannot be used **(Fig. 1)**. Skin being cosmetically important, whatever scar created should be optimum and cosmetically acceptable and so it should be approximated carefully and meticulously.

There are so many methods to suture the skin. Type of the suture and selection of the suture material and needle size depends on the location of the wound, presence of infection and whether primary or secondary suturing. Simple interrupted suture, mattress suture, dermal burial suture, subcuticular suture, etc. are various methods used. Decision taken to use which type depends on the tension required to approximate the wound, size, and type of the wound. Simple and mattress sutures are commonly used **(Fig. 2)**.

## SIMPLE INTERRUPTED SUTURING

It is one of the most commonly used suture to skin, other being simple mattress suture (vertical mattress). It is technically easier; maintains approximation with adequate tension. *Needle is passed perpendicular to the epidermis* traversing in depth across the epidermis and dermis in full thickness; later, it is passed from deeper plane towards and across the skin (dermis and epidermis) on the opposite wound edge. Symmetry should be maintained both in terms of depth and width. Ideally, suture should have flask like configuration with wider dermal part than epidermal part to achieve proper eversion and so that scar wound shall be depressed after healing. Bites at wound edges should be evenly placed; often to prevent the mismatched stepping of the wound edges. Whenever wound tension is needed larger bites should be taken; smaller bites coapt the edges precisely.

If full thickness bites of equidistant are taken, it achieves good apposition.

Usually needle is pierced around 8–10 mm from the wound edge passes across the epidermis, full thickness dermis (wider than epidermis), then opposite side dermis and epidermis; needle curvature can be rotated across all these layers by fluid motion of the wrist by holding and lifting the same and opposite side edges respectively as a single stroke. Pierced needle body on the opposite skin edge is held with forceps or needle holder to remove the needle by rotation movement in the direction of the curvature. If tissue bulk is more, then needle pricks can be taken one after other from same and opposite edges. Knots should be placed on one side of the wound; not over the apposed wound.

It is often also used as a second layer closure of the wound after deeper tissues and dermis are sutured; here small bites are taken from the epidermis only. Simple interrupted sutures are also used in approximating the soft tissues such as muscle, fascia, aponeurosis, and deeper tissues. In circumcision simple interrupted sutures are placed using fine absorbable sutures such as polyglactin or *chromic catgut* (4-0).

*Note:* Olden days surgeons were using straight needle to suture skin and also often while doing bowel anastomosis. Now it is not a common practice.

*Suture material used:* The thinnest suture material should be used; 5-0 in face; 4-0 in upper limbs; 3-0 in trunks and lower limbs. Decision should be taken depending on the anatomical location of the wound, skin/tissue texture and tension. Thinner suture material causes better scar; thicker one may be needed in tension area. Cutting or reverse-cutting needle with monofilament nonabsorbable suture (polypropylene) should be used.

*Depth correcting simple interrupted suturing:* It is used whenever there is disparity in the depth of the edges of the wound. Disparity occurs due to poor apposition of the deeper soft tissues or due to anatomical configuration itself (nasal walls, cheek, and eyelid). Here a shallow needle bite

| Goals of suturing | Factors for selection of the suture material | Ten Commandments in suturing |
|---|---|---|
| • One should be gentle in handling the tissues<br>• Closing the dead space<br>• It should support and strengthen the wounds until healing<br>• Initial healing occurs with type I collagen which has got weak tensile strength and later strong type III collagen forms. So initial period of wound healing needs suture support<br>• It should approximate the wound edges to achieve adequate structural, functional and an aesthetically acceptable<br>• Minimizing the risks of bleeding and infection<br>• To reduce the pain<br>• To achieve linear scar *(Scar is Surgeon's signature)* | • Anatomic location of the wound<br>• Type of the wound<br>• Thickness of the tissue and depth<br>• Tension on the tissue or wound edges<br>• Cosmesis to be achieved | 1. Adequate and proper anesthesia—local/regional/general<br>2. Proper lighting for optimum vision<br>3. Aseptic approach<br>4. Clearing the foreign body in the wound<br>5. Warm saline irrigation of the wound<br>6. Absolute hemostasis<br>7. Minimizing the dead space<br>8. Optimum tension (Tension-free adequate apposition)<br>9. Selection of ideal instruments (needle holder and toothed forceps [type and size of the needle holder is also important]), ideal needle (curvature), ideal type and size of the suture material (Jenkin's Rule)<br>10. Decision taking for type of suturing technique to be used (simple/mattress/continuous/interrupted/or any other types) depending on the type of wound, its tension, depth, contamination, blood supply |

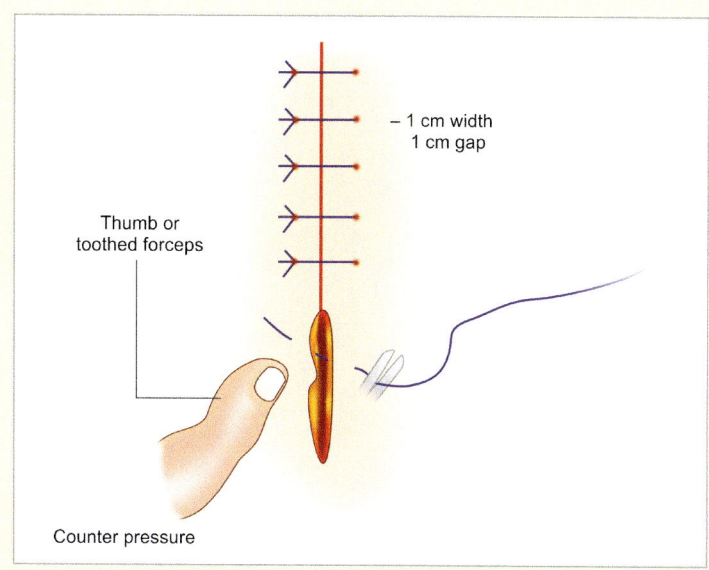

**Fig. 1:** Principles of suturing.

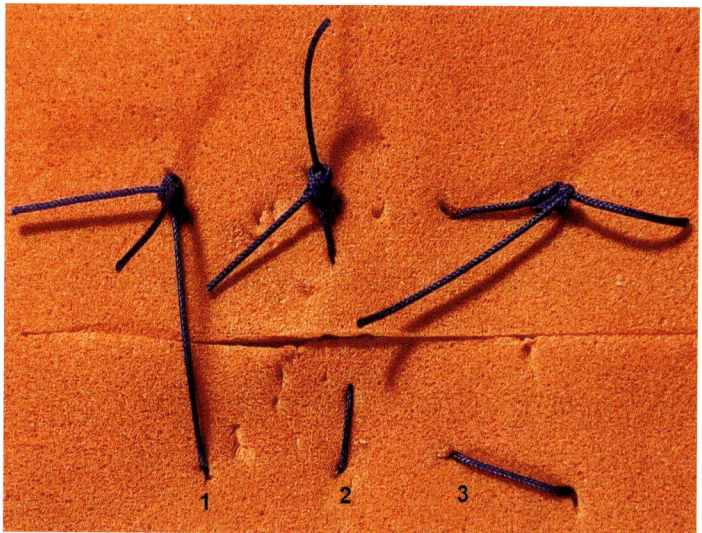

**Fig. 2:** Simple and mattress sutures are commonly used. (1) Simple interrupted suture; (2) Vertical mattress suture; (3) Horizontal mattress suture.

is taken on the side of wound edge which is higher than the opposite side whereas usual deeper bite of dermis is taken on the opposite side wound edge which is lower. Knot is tied very gently to achieve proper apposition and tightened gently to avoid constriction of the overlying epidermis. This suture should be selectively used, not on regular basis **(Figs. 3A to C)**.

*Problems:* Wound inversion can occur easily resulting in *wound gaping* or *depressed poor scar*. Stitch abscess formation, track marks, and necrosis can occur. While taking bites, needle may penetrate small vessel leading to *bleeding* which often may not stop by mere pressure. In such situation, additional bites of suturing at the bleeding area with tight (firm) knotting will stop bleeding but this indirect ligation may lead into poor scar eventually; alternatively few already placed sutures can be removed to identify the bleeding vessel which can be individually ligated using absorbable fine sutures or fulgurated using bipolar cautery.

*Advantages:* It is quick and hemostatic; easier to remove; and performed in urgent situation.

*Simple interrupted fascial suture:* It is used in abdominal wall like in closure of *McBurney* incision by taking about 5-8 mm of tissue bite.

*Simple everting suture:* It is used in skin. Bites at deeper plane should be wider than superficial plane. Edges should be everted once this stitch is placed.

## SIMPLE RUNNING SUTURING

It is used as second layer continuous epidermal closure suture, once deeper layer is closed or often in lengthy wounds for quick closure but after proper closure of deeper layers. It is also useful in fixing skin grafts to recipient edge using continuous fine absorbable/nonabsorbable suture material.

Beginning of suturing is similar to simple interrupted suture; after placing knot, leading needle side is not cut; instead repetitive, equidistant, uniform parallel bites, and throws are taken placing intersecting parallel suture lines; once last throw is taken suture material loop is kept loosely on side opposite to the final needle bite side and suture material is tied using instrument knot. Here all loops of suture are placed in succession.

*Drawbacks:* Loosening of suture material can happen compromising the integrity of the entire suture line as it rests entirely

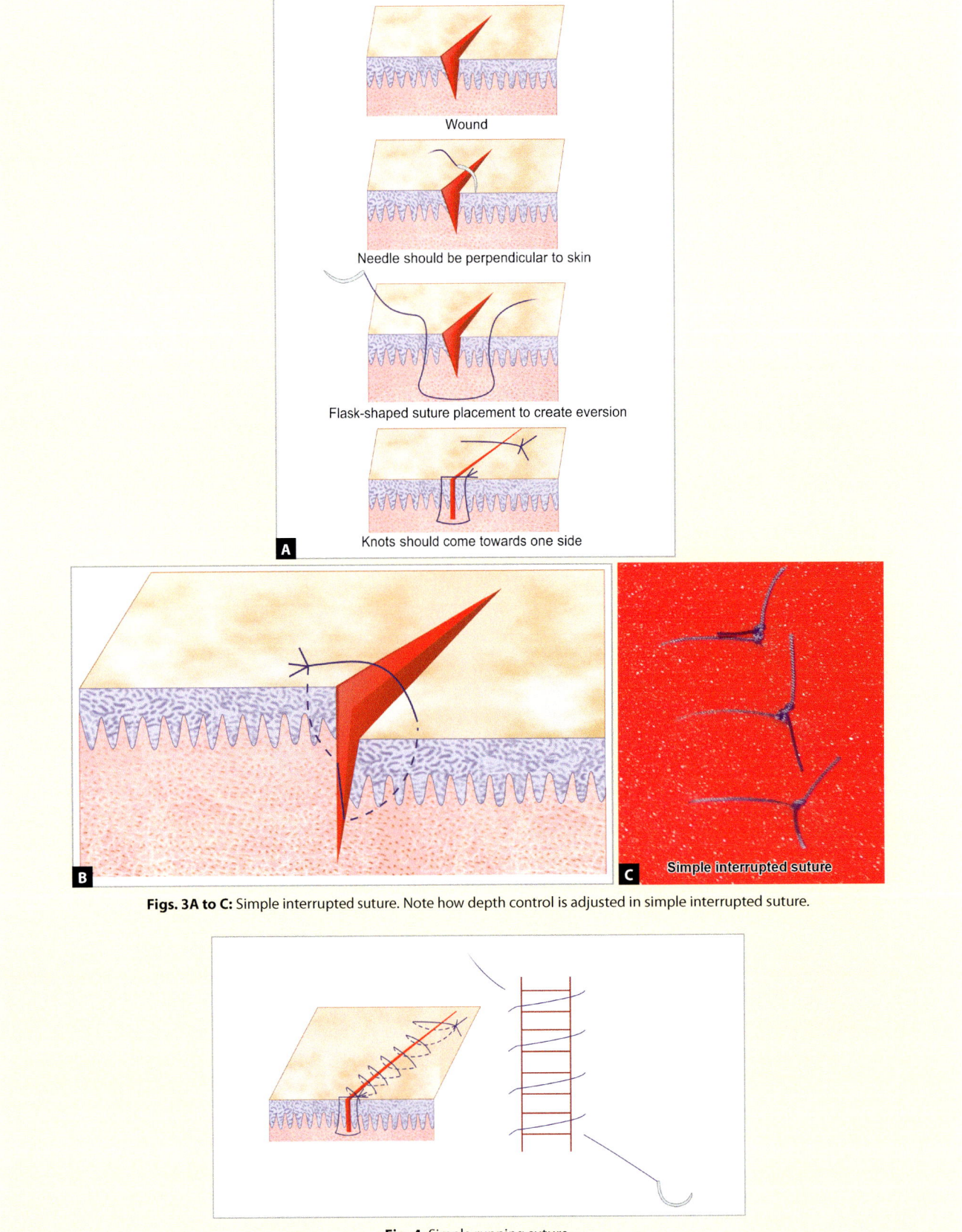

**Figs. 3A to C:** Simple interrupted suture. Note how depth control is adjusted in simple interrupted suture.

**Fig. 4:** Simple running suture.

on two end knots. Inversion, track marks, wound breakdown, and puckering of the suture line are the problems. This suture is usually removed early and so might cause wound disruption at a later period **(Figs. 4 and 5)**.

*Running locked suturing:* Simple running suture can be unlocked or locked. After tying first knot after first bite, each running continuous suture is locked by passing through the preceding loop and tightened; end knot is tied by placing the knot to the last loop. After each looping, assistant should hold the loop away with some tension to achieve uniformity in tension and locking. Needle bites from the each edges of the wound should be taken from equidistant and same level to achieve parallel looping and locking. But integrity of the suture depends on mainly two end knots. It will provide equal and better tension along the length of the wound. It is hemostatic also and creates eversion of the wound edge. It is used in traumatic wounds as it is hemostatic; in patients who are on aspirin therapy. Track marks, necrosis, superficial nerve damage, and inversion still can occur. Suture should be removed early here.

*Continuous over and over simple suture:* It is continuous suture used in peritoneum, fascia, and aponeurosis. Vicryl is used usually. *Continuous over and over suture*—it is continuous sutures taken at equidistant. It should not be very tight as more tightening may cause strangulation of the wound edge; it may cause bunching of the wound; but it saves time.

*Continuous locking sutures (continuous blanket sutures/Ford sutures):* It is not commonly used in skin. It is used in closure of fascial layer. It holds well and is hemostatic. It is commonly used in closure of rectus sheath. Nonabsorbable suture material is usually used. It does not cause bunching of the wound **(Figs. 6 and 7)**.

*Continuous "mass closure"*—using 1 or 0 monofilament nonabsorbable suture material commonly used in closure of abdominal incisions especially midline. Bites are taken at 1 cm width from wound edge; with each bite at 1 cm interval. Single strand or loop suture material can be used for this. This method is commonly used. Often in between closure knots are placed to prevent suture getting loosened. It is ended by knot on loop or by Aberdeen knot **(Fig. 8)**.

The suture material runs intracutaneously on one side (opposite side) of the wound.

*Note:* Jenkin's rule—length of the suture material used is 4 times the length of the wound.

## VERTICAL MATTRESS SUTURE (DONATI/ALLGÖWER-DONATI SUTURING)

**Vertical mattress (Donati) suture:** It is a modification of simple suture wherein two bites are taken from each edge of the wound creating one deep suture to achieve optimum wound tension another superficial to create eversion of the edge. It is most commonly used suture in surgical practice. Needle is passed at 90° from

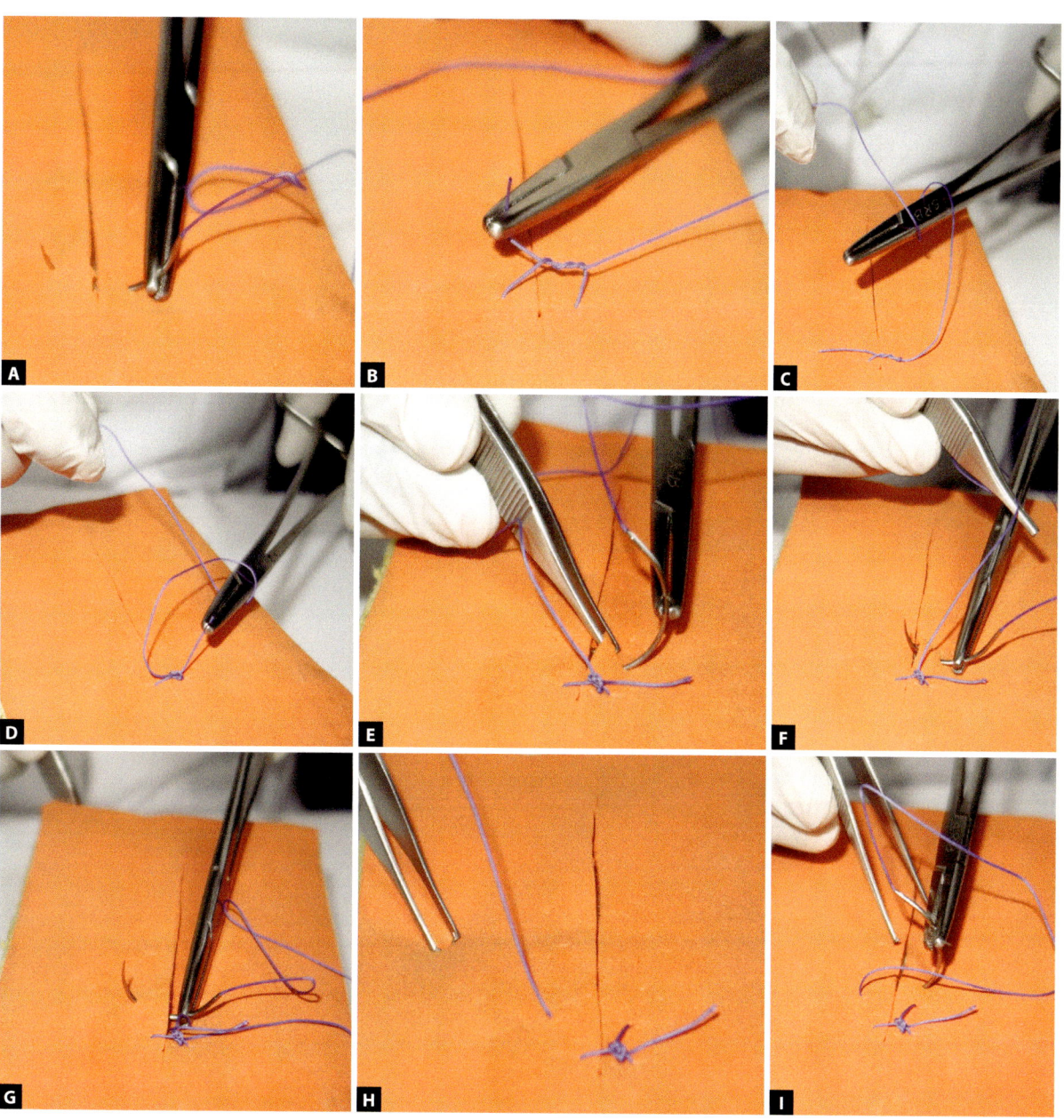

**Figs. 5A to I**

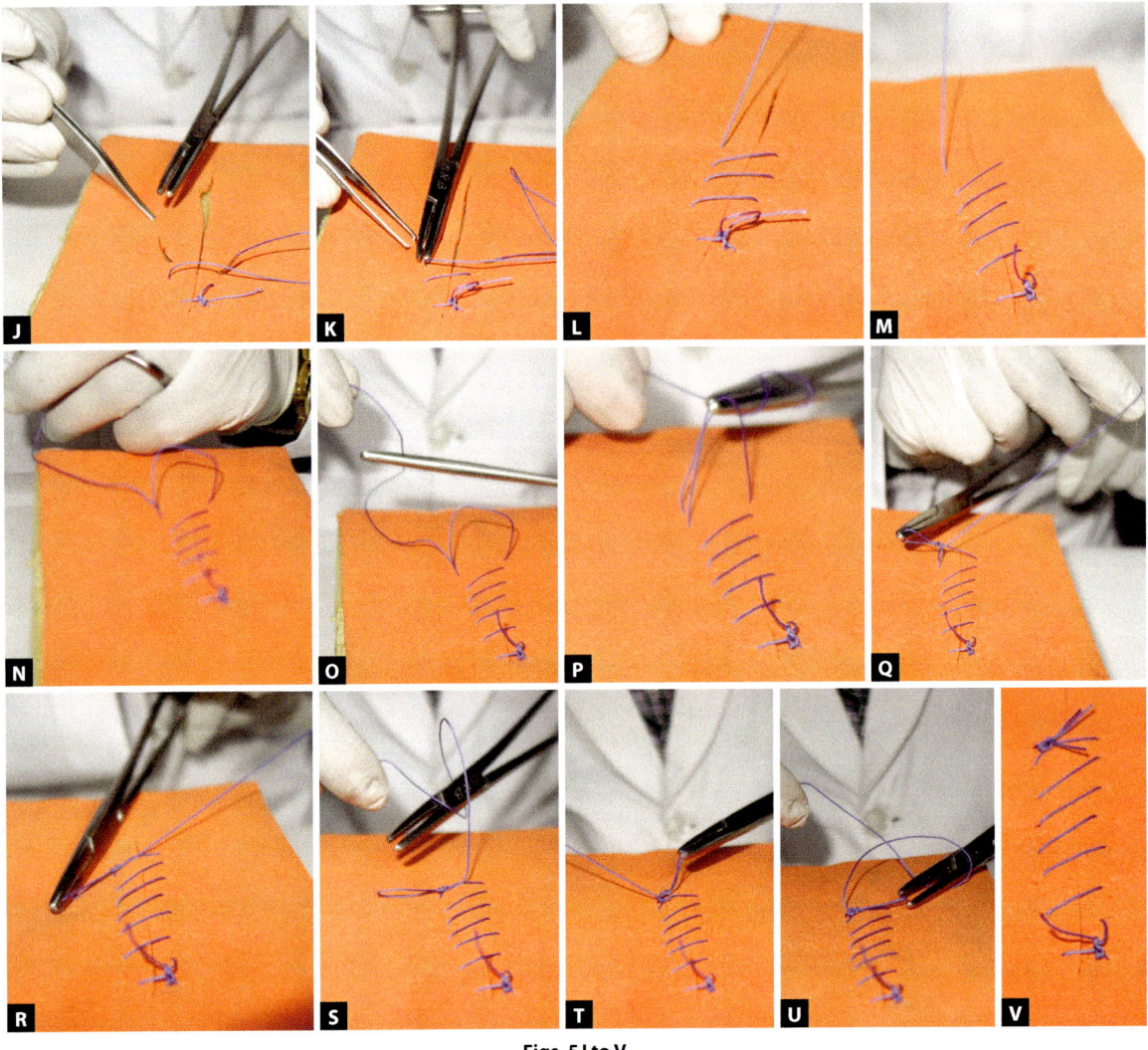

**Figs. 5J to V**

**Figs. 5A to V:** Simple continuous suture with loop knot at the end.

skin across towards depth of the wound 5–6 mm from the wound edge; needle is rotated toward opposite edge from depth to epidermis again keeping the exit point at same line and distant of 5–6 mm; needle is grasped again; using backhand motion needle bite is taken from the opposite side edge around 2–3 mm distant and is passed superficially underneath; bite is taken from depth to skin from the same side to come out to place the knot. It is also called as *far-far and near-near suture* as first entry and exit points are far; eventual entry and exit points are near. Here suture material will not traverse through the surface of the wound. It is useful in areas of natural inversion like creases.

*Drawbacks:* It takes more time to place precise vertical mattress suture. Wound edges may be open due to more eversion. So, often additional simple sutures may require to be placed to superficial part of the wound. Removal is technically difficult; often deeper portion may be left behind the skin **(Figs. 9 to 11)**.

*Short hand vertical mattress:* Here first *near-near superficial bites* are taken; then *far-far deeper bites* are taken. Otherwise final outcome is exactly same; only order of taking bites is exactly reverse of standard technique **(Figs. 12 and 13)**.

*All-Gower's technique:* It is half buried vertical mattress. Needle is passed from far entry point to deeper plane on the same side; from the depth on the opposite side toward and within the margin of the opposite wound edge across the deeper tissue and dermal bite is taken as half buried suture on the opposite edge; further needle bite is taken from the edge of the same side from within out as near suture to exit on the same side of the skin to create half buried vertical mattress perfectly. Here only one entry and one exit points are present on one side of the wound edge only **(Figs. 14A to J)**. The suture material runs intracutaneously on one side (opposite side) of the wound.

*Loop vertical mattress locking suture (loop mattress suture):* It is similar like vertical mattress (far-far and near-near type); but after the last near suture placing, needle with leading suture is looped on the opposite side loop of the suture allowing to pass the suture across the wound edge surface; finally knot is tied on the same side to the trail end of the suture material. It achieves very good wound apposition with reduction in the tension over the suture material **(Figs. 15 and 16)**.

*Far-near and near-far modified vertical mattress suture (pulley suture):* Needle bite is taken for far suture 5–6 mm from the ipsilateral wound edge to pierce into deeper plane; from the deeper plane near suture needle bite on the opposite edge of the wound 2–3 mm from the corresponding (contralateral) edge towards skin surface is taken as exit bite; from here suture material is crossed to ipsilateral side to take near bite 2–3 mm from the wound edge as ipsilateral near bite; lastly from the deeper plane far bite from inside out on the contralateral side is taken as far exit bite; leading end of the suture material is tied on to the trailing end on the ipsilateral side to create two surface loops on the wound surface which completes the pulley vertical mattress suture **(Figs. 17 and 18)**.

***Running vertical mattress suture:*** It is running vertical mattress suture to create everting edge of the wound; it is done after suturing of deeper layer. It is used in genitalia and lacerated wound.

> **Vertical mattress suture (Stewart):** Deep bite is taken from one edge; passed through deeper part of opposite edge and brought out on the opposite edge surface; again close to the superficial margin of opposite side bite is taken and is passed through similar edge of same side to bring out as mattress suture.

***Percutaneous vertical mattress suture (Haneke-Marini suture):*** It is modified buried vertical mattress suture. It is used in situations wherein there is difficulty in placing buried sutures such as in scalp, leg, etc. It is vertical mattress in reverse direction. It is not commonly used. Absorbable suture (4-5-0) is used for this suture. Suture bite is taken from deep dermis toward skin outside; bite is again taken from very close to exit point or through the same exit point to exit through the ipsilateral wound edge; again bite is taken as backhand movement from contralateral skin edge from inside out; through this closer to this exit point on contralateral side bite is taken to reach deep dermis to meet and place a buried knot in the depth using instrument tie.

## HORIZONTAL MATTRESS SUTURE

*Horizontal mattress suture:* It is not commonly used in skin. It is often used in retention sutures (tension sutures), fascial closure, and ventral hernia repair, to achieve hemostasis. Here bite is taken like a square with two time bites on each side one below the other. It is simple interrupted sutures with additional parallel bites taken in reverse. It everts the skin edges of wounds under tension **(Figs. 19 and 20)**.

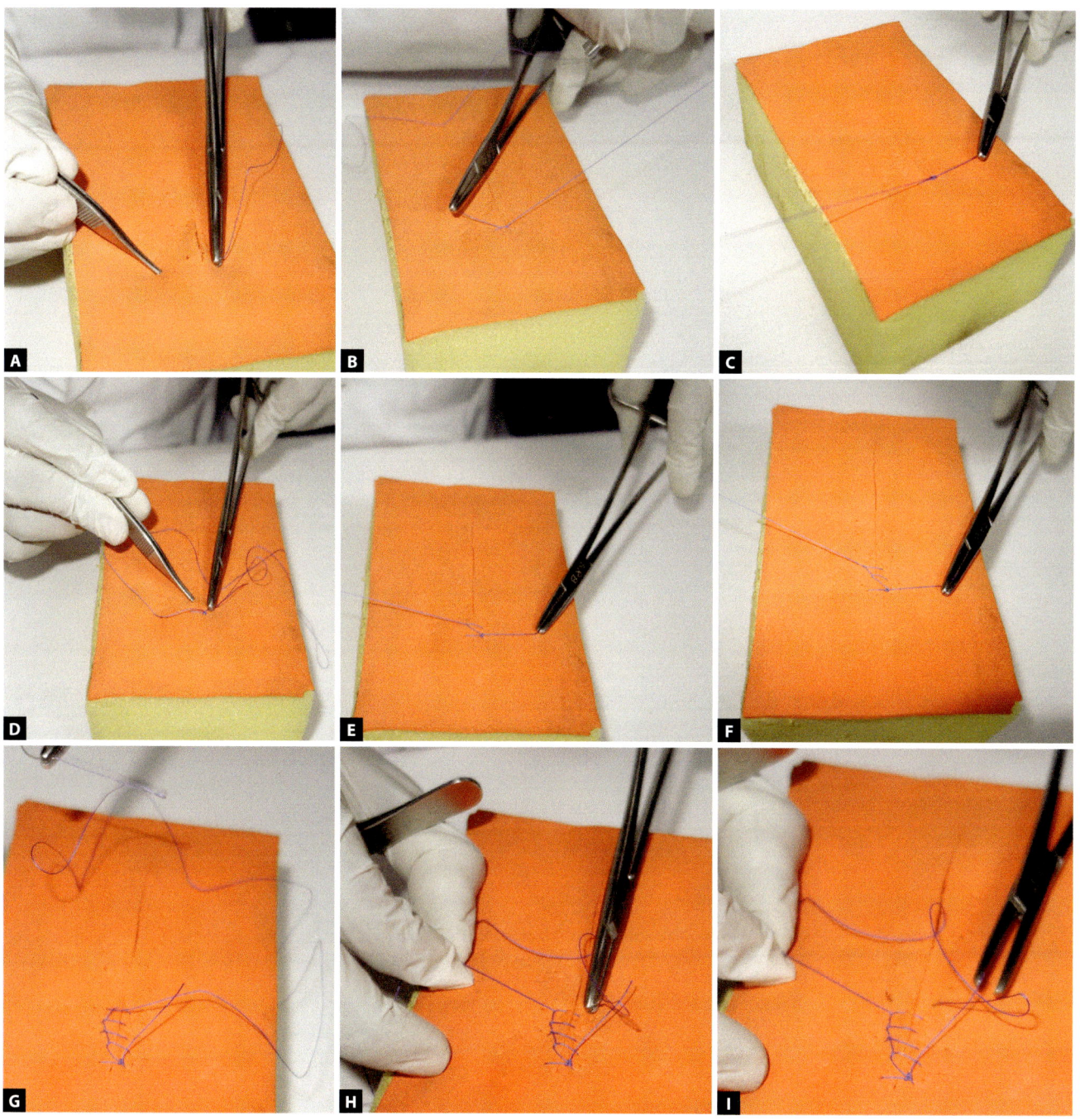

**Figs. 6A to I**

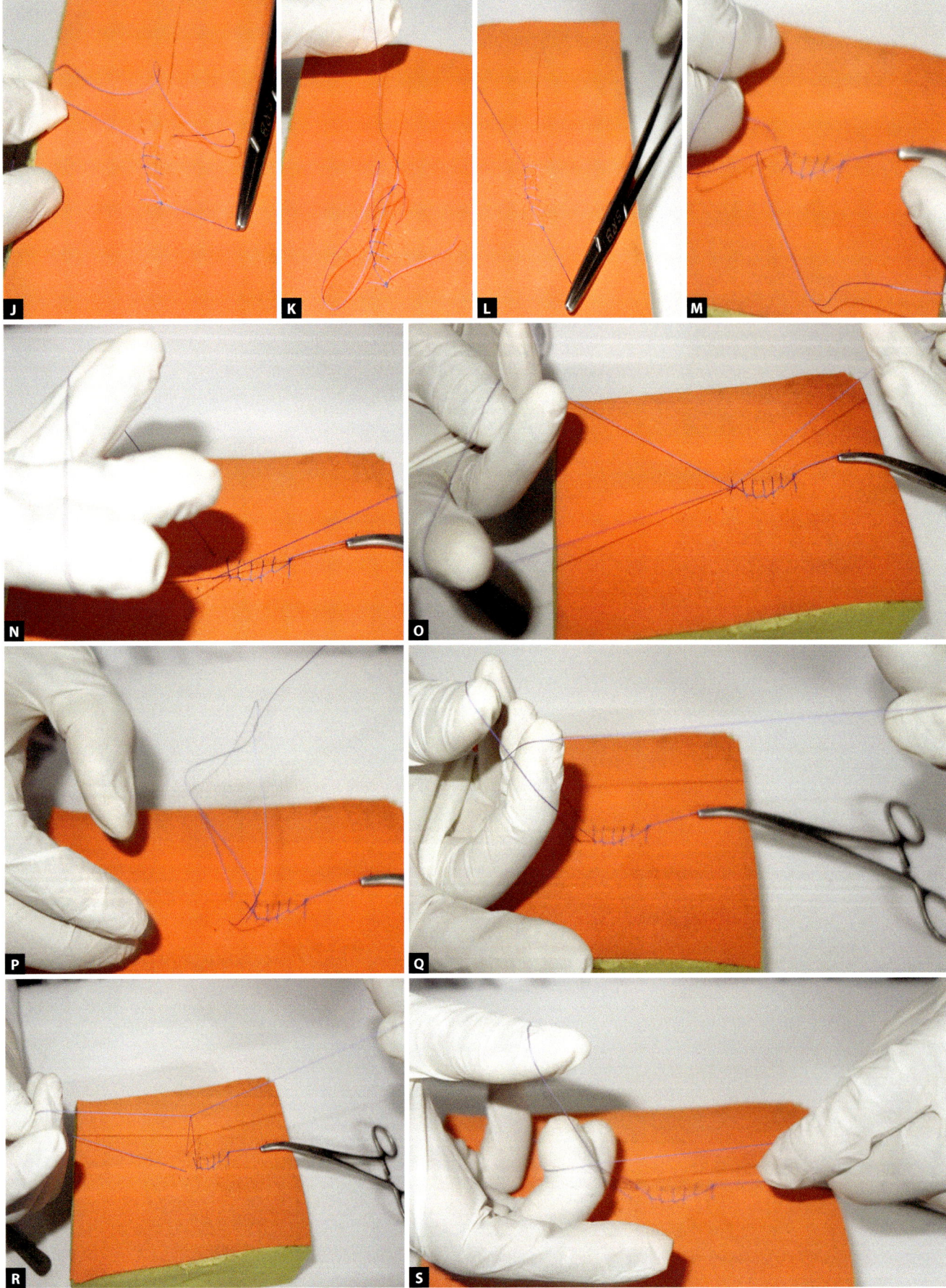

Figs. 6J to S

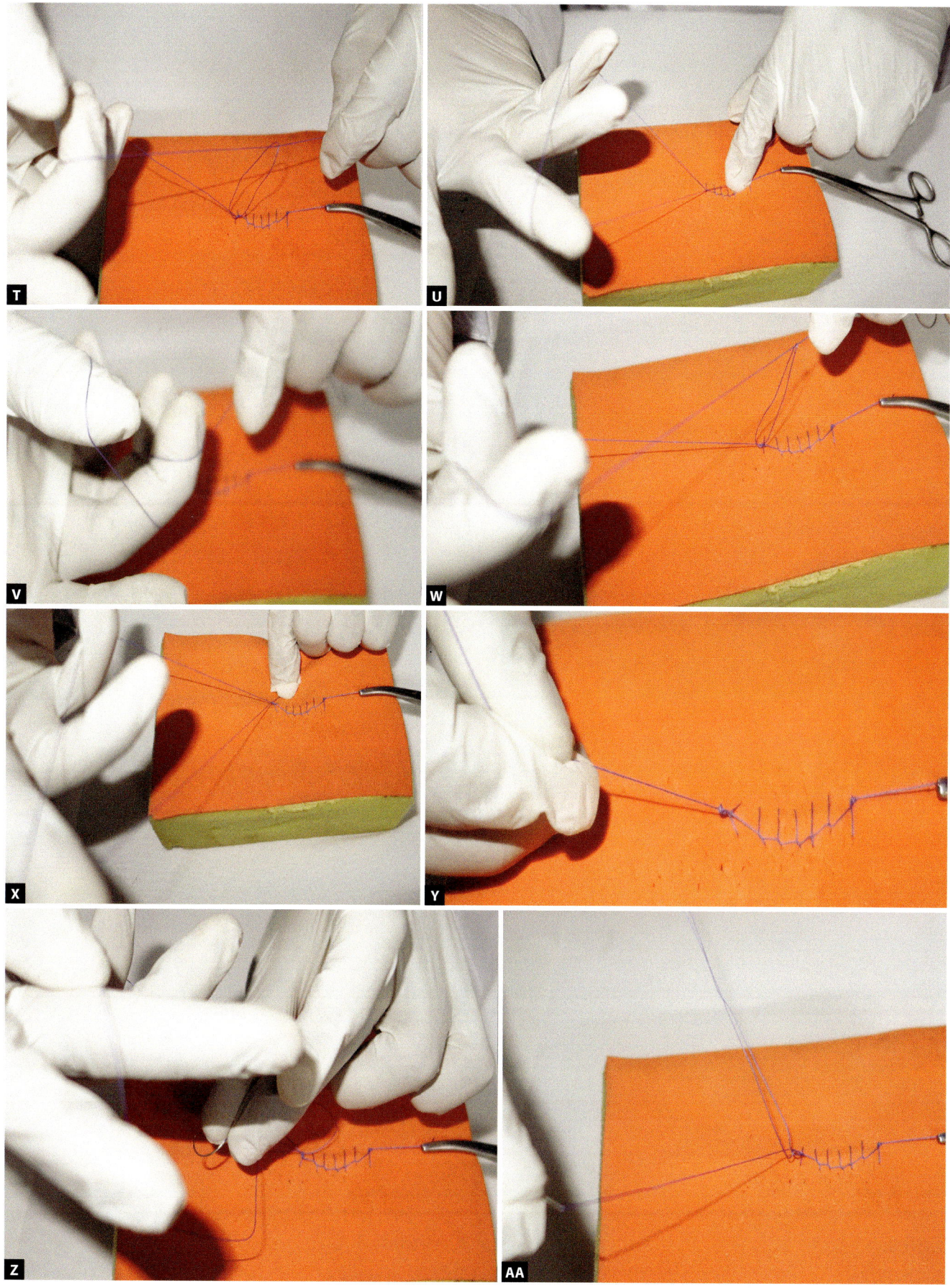

**Figs. 6T to AA**

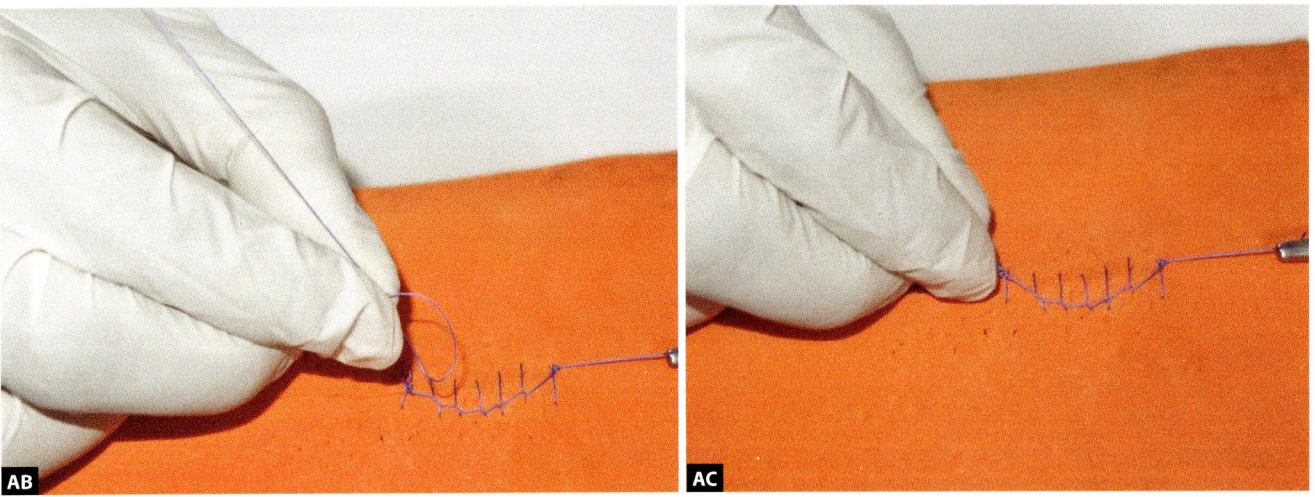

**Figs. 6AB and AC**
**Figs. 6A to AC:** Continuous locking suture with Aberdeen knot.

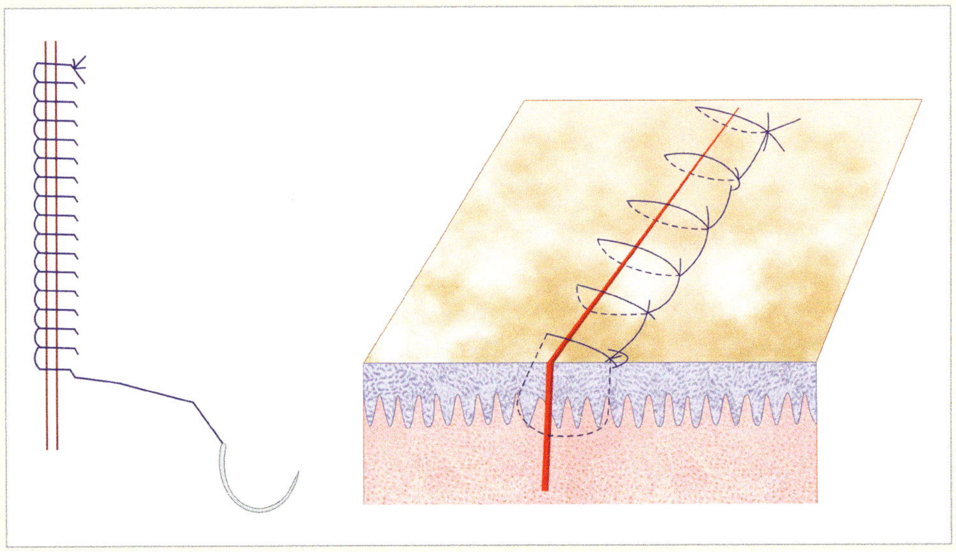

**Fig. 7:** Continuous locking suture.

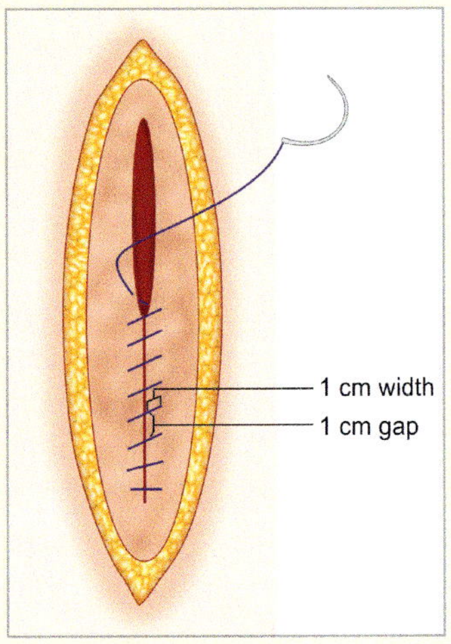

**Fig. 8:** Continuous mass closure of the abdomen.

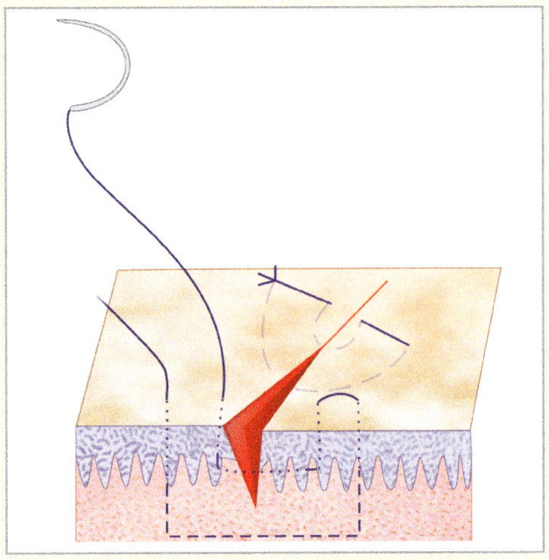

**Fig. 9:** Vertical mattress suture (Stewart).

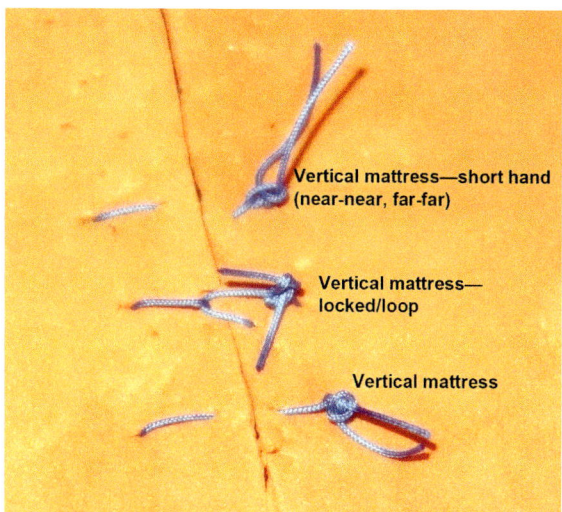

**Fig. 10:** Different types of vertical mattress sutures usually practiced.

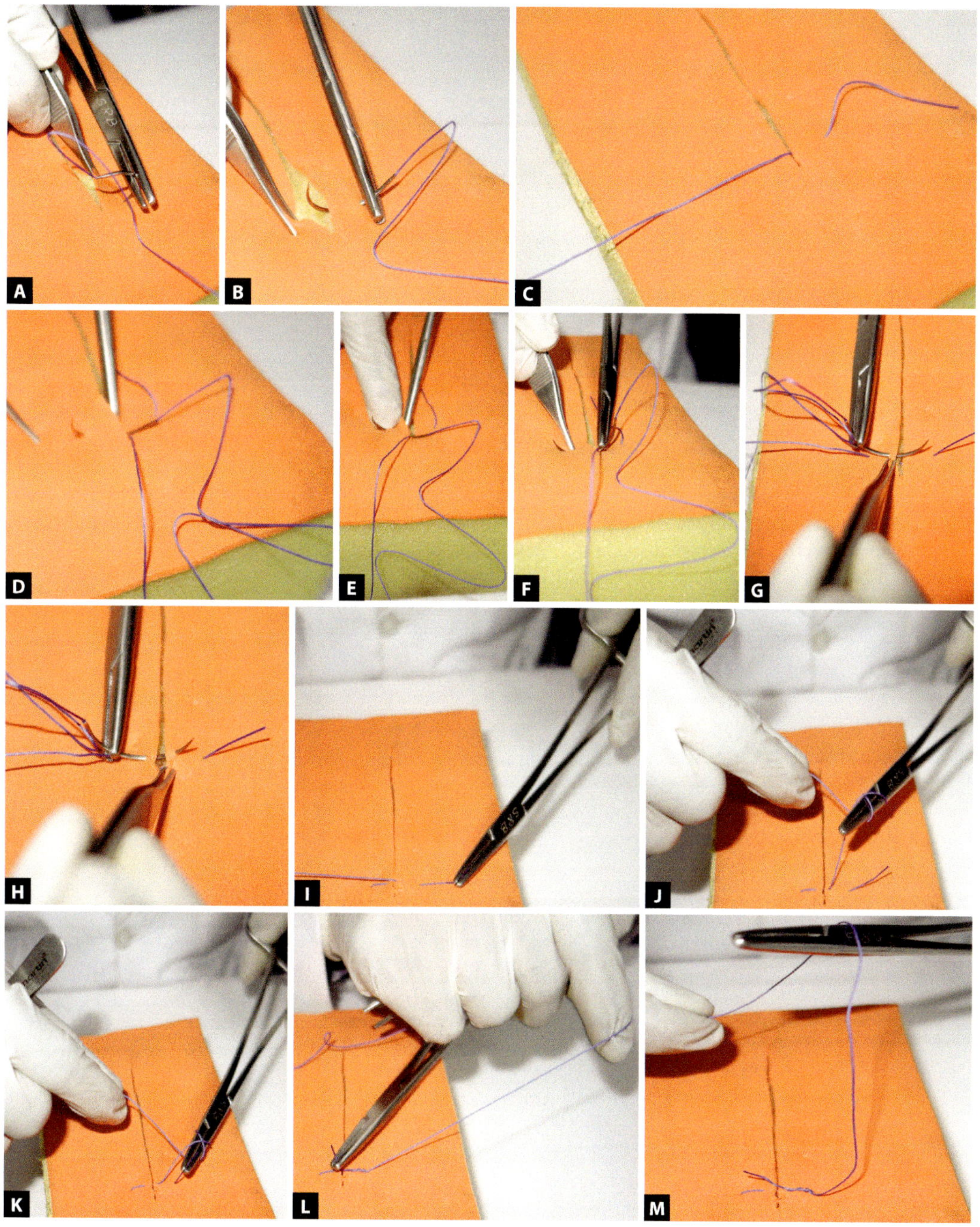

**Figs. 11A to M**

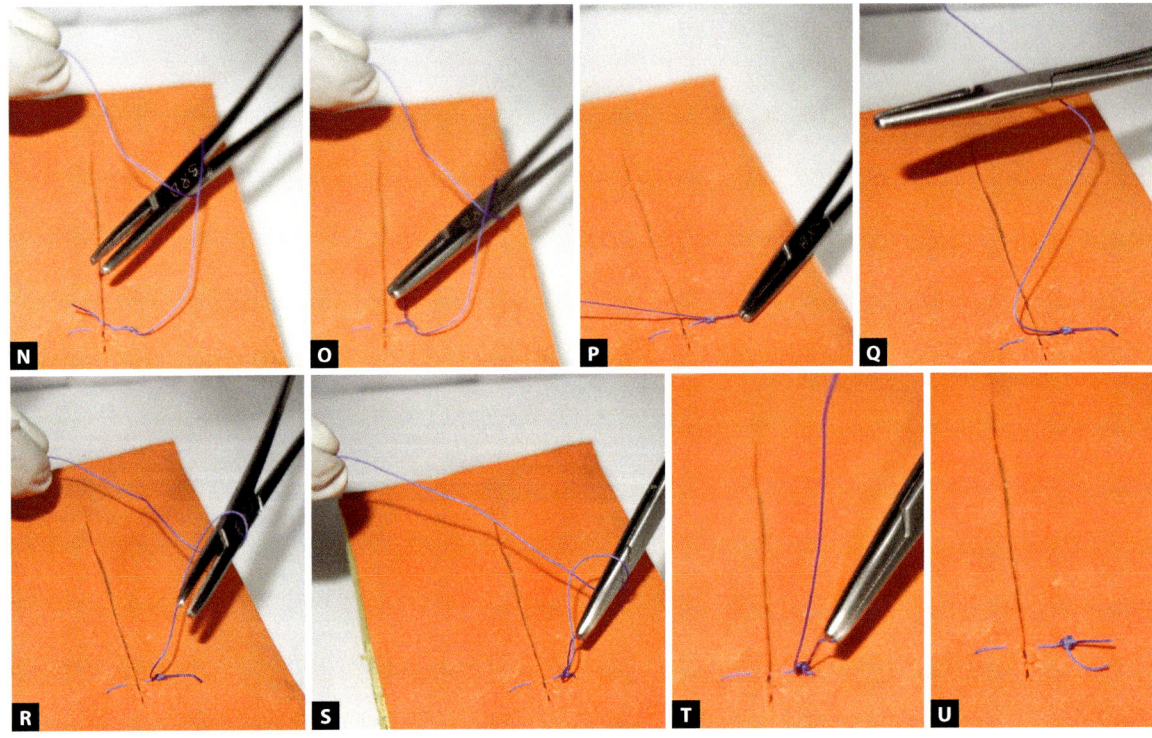

**Figs. 11N to U**

**Figs. 11A to U:** Technique of vertical mattress suture placement.

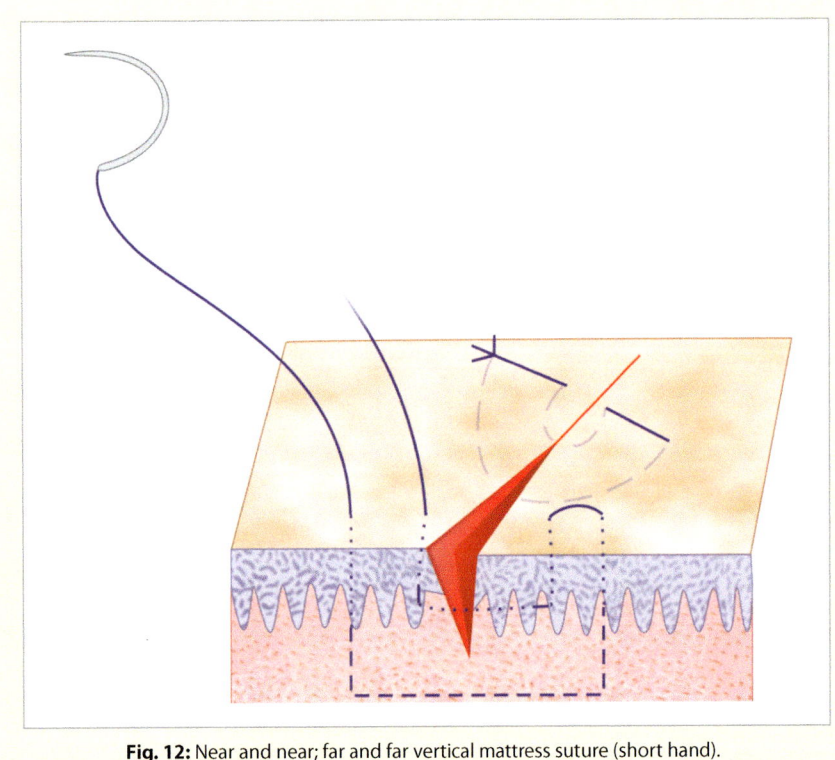

**Fig. 12:** Near and near; far and far vertical mattress suture (short hand).

*Drawback of mattress suture:* There is increased risk of track marks, tissue strangulation, and improper wound healing.

*Locking horizontal mattress suture:* Here after taking far bites of two edges loop is kept loose while taking second far bite of the opposite edge; once second far bite of the ipsilateral (first) edge is done needle with suture is passed through the loose loop kept and tightened to place the suture. This creates better eversion and wound edge apposition. This later allows suture removal easier preventing the knot and suture getting buried in the epidermis **(Fig. 21)**.

*Inverting horizontal mattress suture:* It is useful in apposing natural creases like in eyelid and crease lines. It gives moderate tissue tension and hold without compressing vascularity. Track marks are less common. Wound inversion is good **(Fig. 22)**.

## Other Mattress Sutures

Different modifications of mattress sutures are used even though they are not that commonly used. Examples are locking horizontal mattress suture, inverting horizontal mattress suture; running horizontal mattress suture; running locking horizontal mattress suture; cruciate mattress suture; running oblique mattress suture; double locking horizontal mattress suture; running diagonal mattress suture; running vertical mattress suture; hybrid mattress suture, etc. **(Figs. 23A and B)**.

## SUBCUTICULAR SUTURE

It is used in skin closure. Needle bite is taken initially at one corner; it is continued by taking bites at the white dermis on each side alternatively to reach the other end of the wound; which is then brought out through the corner of the wound. Usually absorbable polyglycolic acid/poliglecaprone (Monocryl) is used (4-6-0) with curved cutting needle. It is difficult to place subcuticular

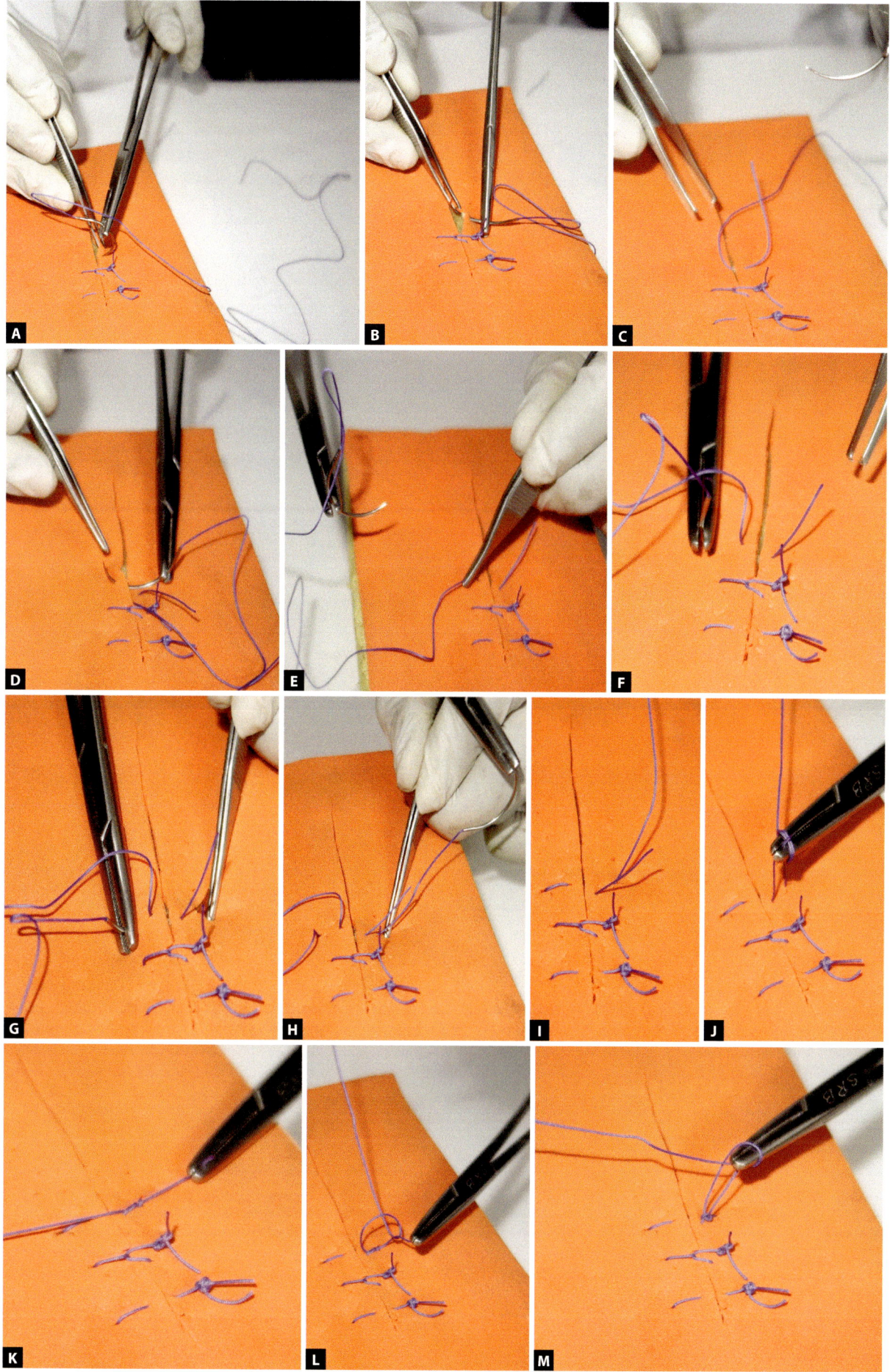

**Figs. 13A to M:** Near and near, far and far vertical mattress suture.

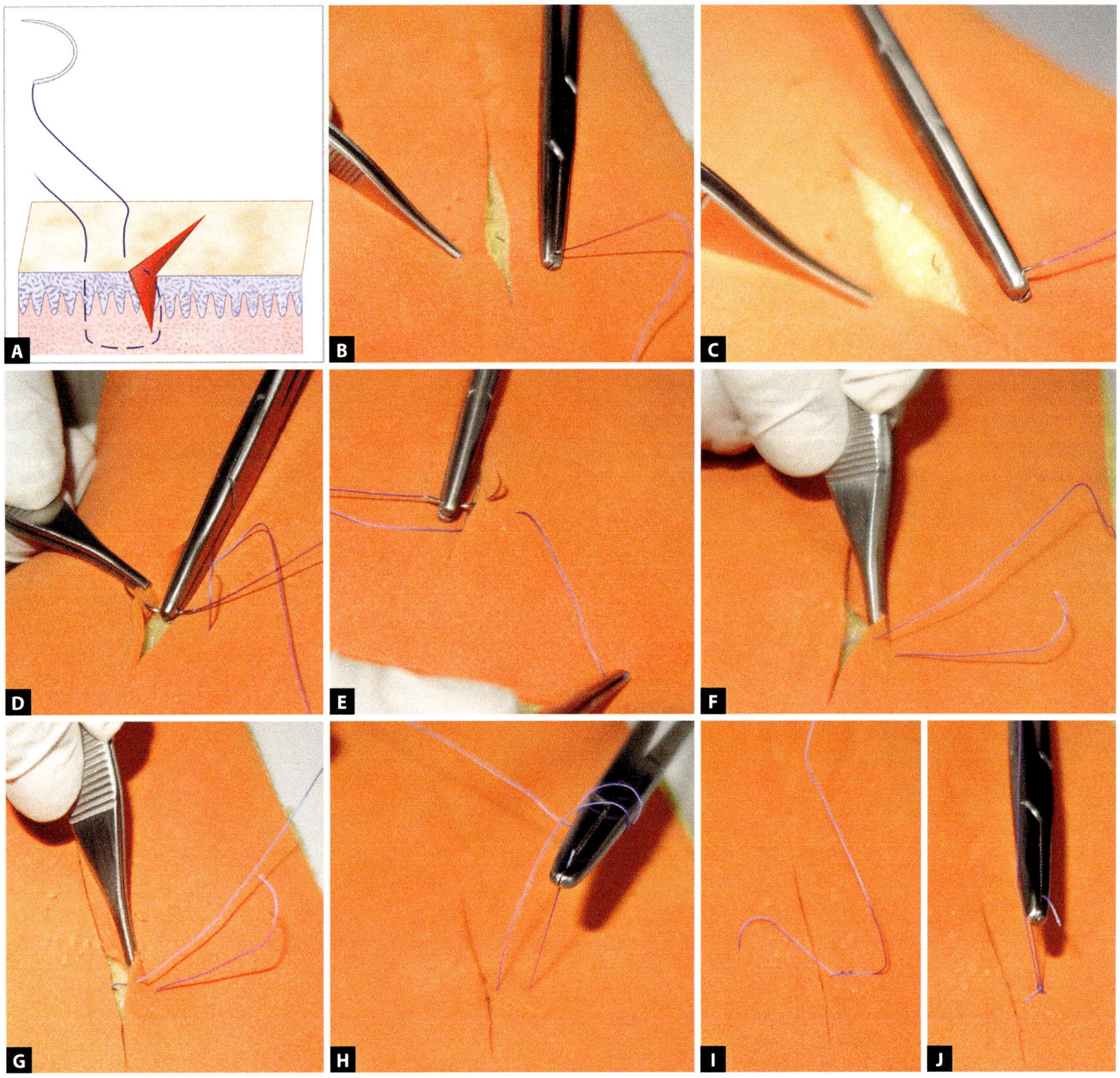

**Figs. 14A to J:** Vertical mattress—Allgöwer suture technique.

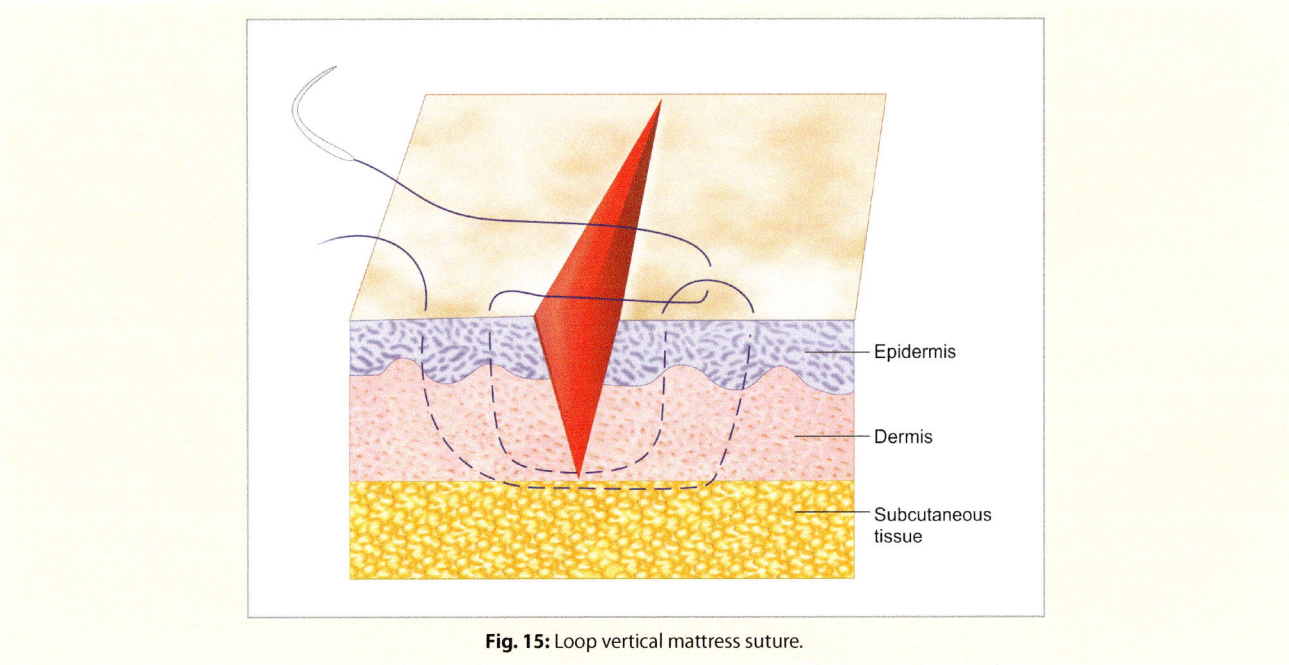

**Fig. 15:** Loop vertical mattress suture.

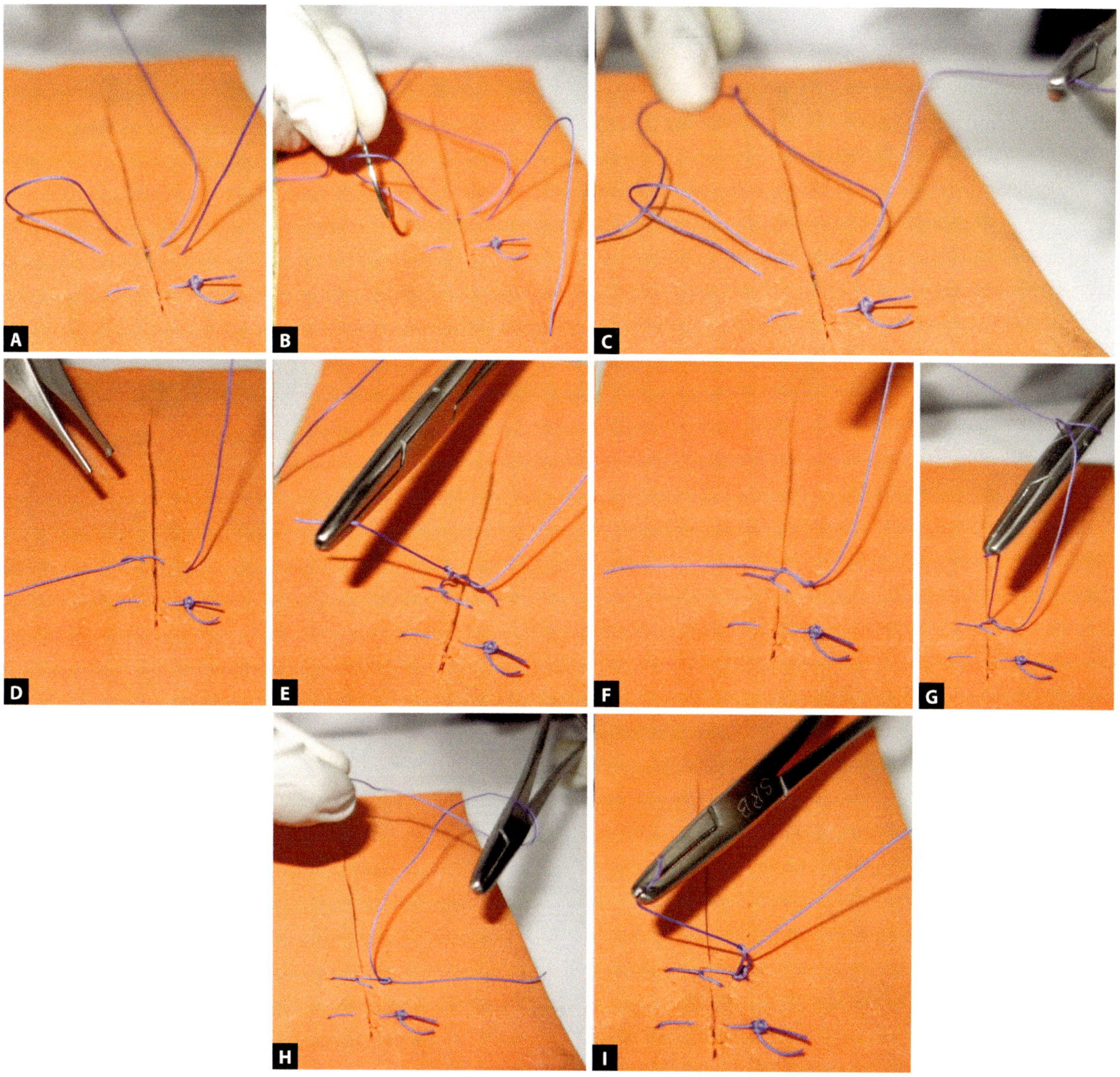

# Skin and Soft Tissue Suturing

**Figs. 16A to I:** Locking vertical mattress suture.

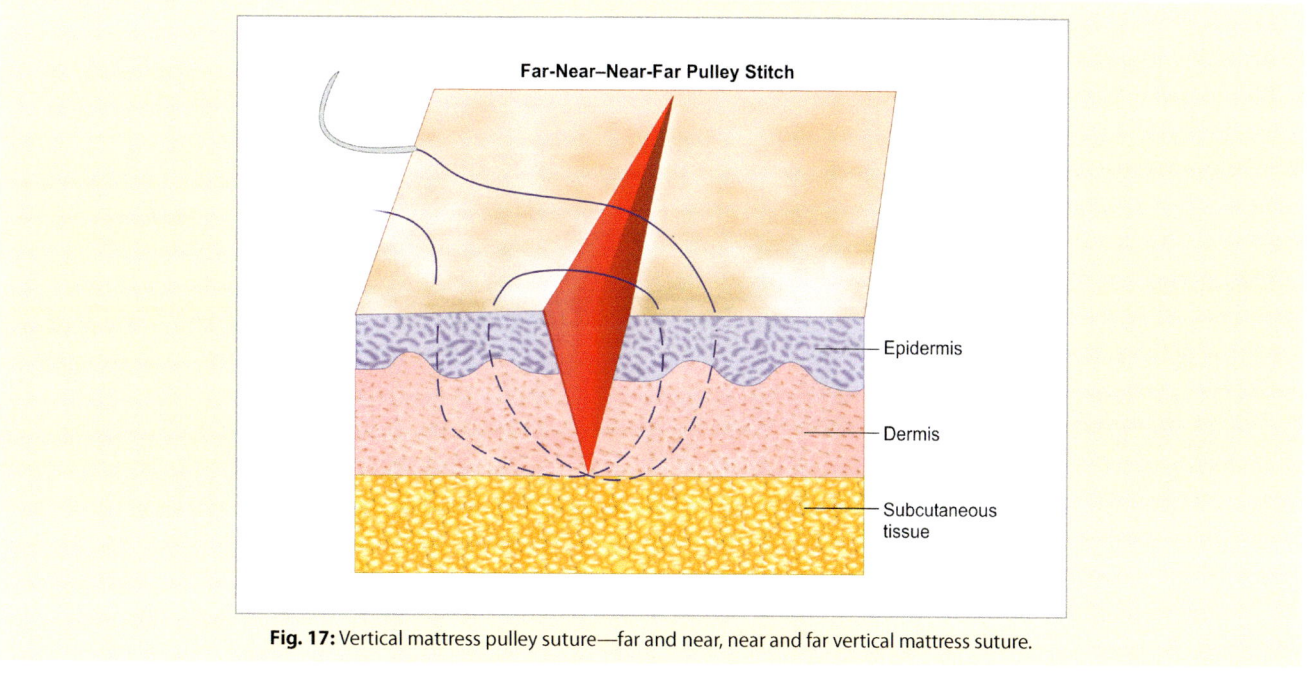

**Fig. 17:** Vertical mattress pulley suture—far and near, near and far vertical mattress suture.

sutures using round body needle. Cutting needle is ideal. Absorbable suture is not removed. Nonabsorbable monofilament suture can also be used. Its ends are left long or tied loosely over gauze. It is removed in 10 days. Often there may be difficulty in pulling out the sutures. Subcuticular suture gives cosmetically better scar. But if sutures thicker than 3-0 is used it will cause inflammatory reaction in the apposed wound causing no cosmetic benefit. Subcuticular sutures should not be used in trauma, infective areas, and emergency surgeries. There is controversy whether it has got advantage over interrupted sutures using fine material except in avoiding (in absorbable subcuticular)/ easier (nonabsorbable subcuticular) suture removal.

It is based on strong dermal suture which keeps the epidermis in apposed position. It can be used only when there is no wound tension and when dermis is thick and strong. It cannot be used in places such as eyelid and skin with thin dermis. There are several ways of beginning and ending the subcuticular suture. When absorbable suture is used; at the wound corner bite is taken over the dermis and knot is placed; tail end is cut close to the knot; bite is taken from ipsilateral dermis for 2-5 mm apart parallel to the epidermis; further bite is taken from contralateral dermis of similar type. Alternate ipsilateral and contralateral parallel bites are taken through dermis until it reaches to opposite wound angle (apex). Nonabsorbable suture when used (monofilament polypropylene) first bite is taken 2-3 mm away from the angle of the wound which is brought out of the apex of the wound (angle) through dermis (dermis is pale, tough, whitish structure) and from here, it is passed through alternate parallel 3-5 mm dermal bites until it is reaches towards opposite angle/apex wherein it is

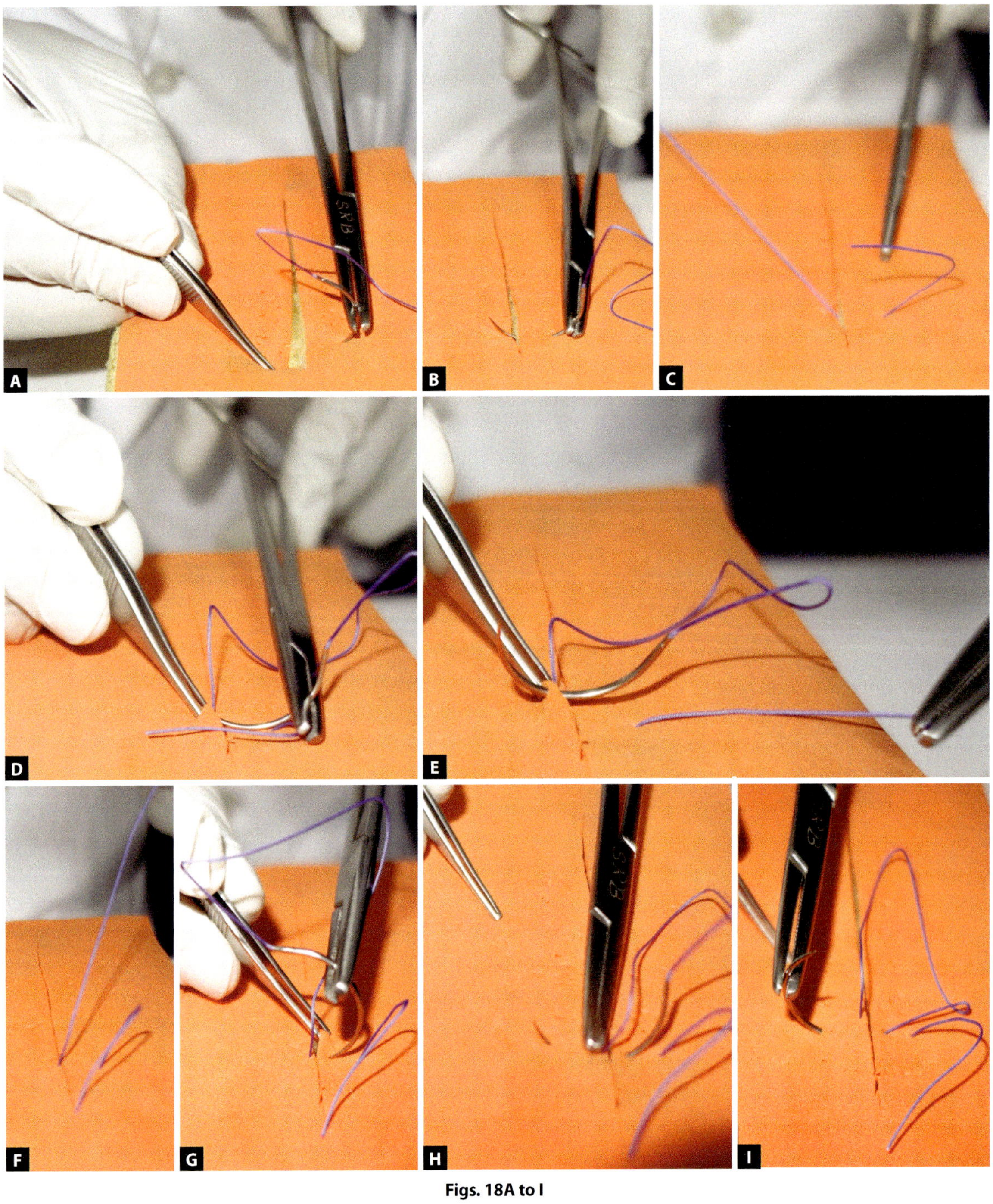

**Figs. 18A to I**

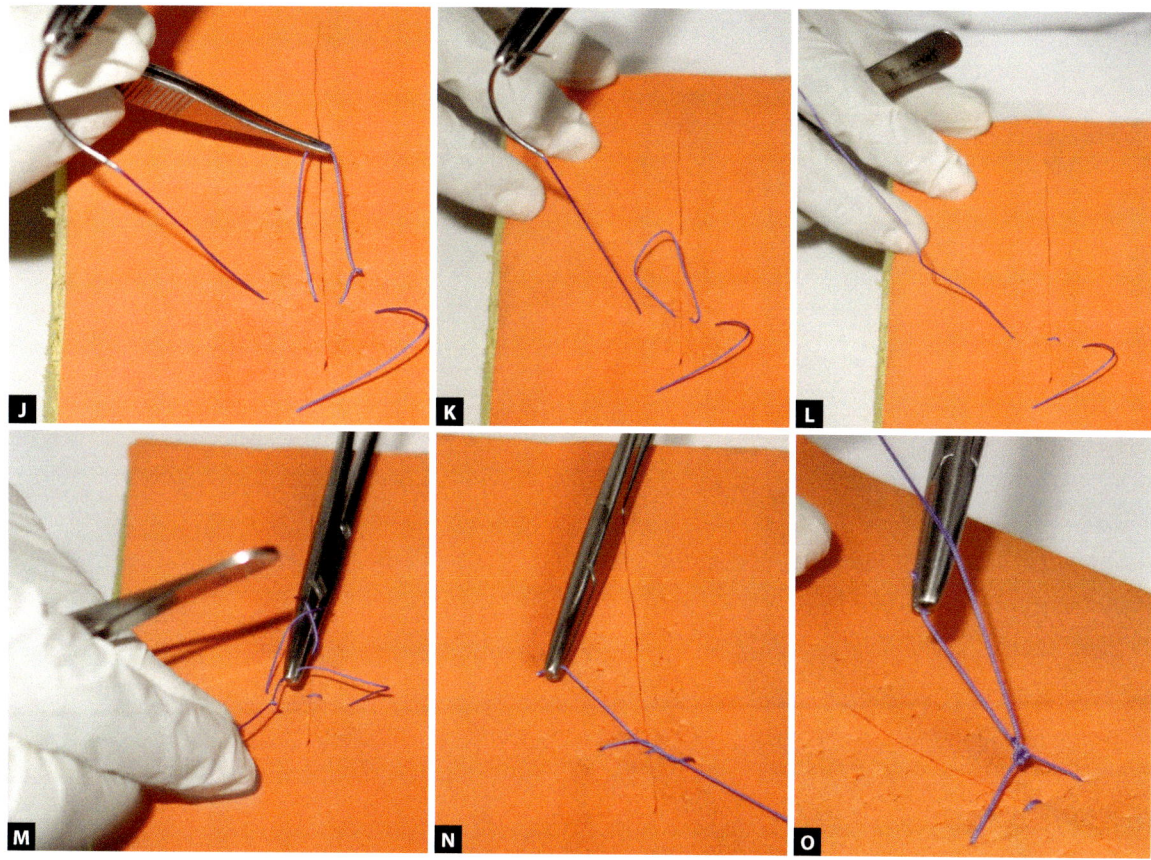

**Figs. 18J to O**

**Fig. 18A to O:** Vertical mattress—far and near; near and far—pulley suture.

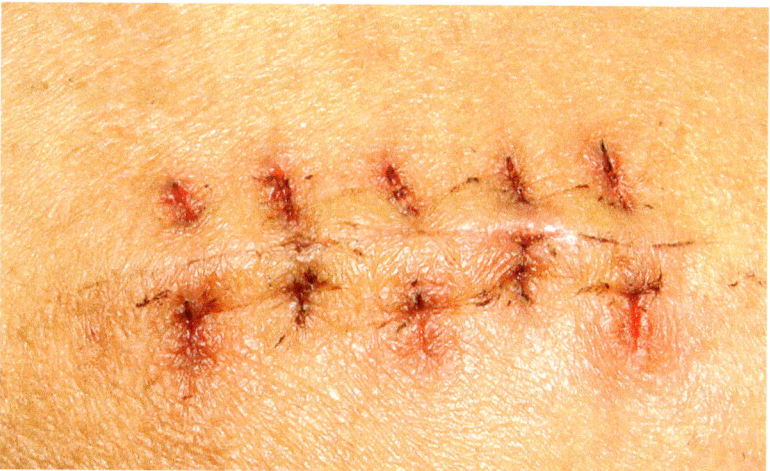

**Fig. 19:** Scar of interrupted sutures—vertical mattress sutures.

brought out through the skin 3–5 mm from the angle.

Subcuticular suture is ended in absorbable suture by placing two throws knot at the angle in the dermis or by two loop—Aberdeen knot. Often it is brought out through the apex and suture is cut flush with the skin. In nonabsorbable suture, since it needs to be removed by pulling the suture gently from one angle of the wound after 7 days, both ends should be kept long so that smooth removal can be facilitated. Both ends can be tied over the wound like a bow with a gauze placement underneath over the apposed wound. While removal suture is cut at one angle and is pulled out away from the opposite angle.

*Problems with subcuticular suture are:* (1) Crumpling of the edges of the wound with wound inversion at epidermis can occur; (2) Foreign body reaction in the dermis can occur, when absorbable suture is left in the wound edge; (3) Track formation in the dermis which may create a poor linear scar even though it avoids bite marks on the edges; and (4) When nonabsorbable suture is used often removal is difficult **(Figs. 24A and B)**.

## OTHER METHODS OF TISSUE APPROXIMATION IN VARIOUS PLACES

### Hemostatic Figure of Eight Suture

It is basically used for hemostasis. It is used in circumcision to ligate frenular artery, bleeders withdrawn into the soft tissues. Vicryl or polypropylene (2-0/3-0) is used **(Fig. 25)**.

### Three-point Suture

It is used in suturing triangular flap/flaps to have correct apposition. Dermal bites should be at the same levels on both edges **(Fig. 26)**.

### Purse-string Suture

It is used wherein center part of the tissue or wound needs to get buried off. After open appendicectomy, appendix stump is buried using purse-string seromuscular sutures around the stump on the cecum **(Fig. 27)**.

### Interrupted Cruciate Suture

It is two bites which are taken from each side to create a cruciate mattress suture. It is used, whenever there is less tension in the

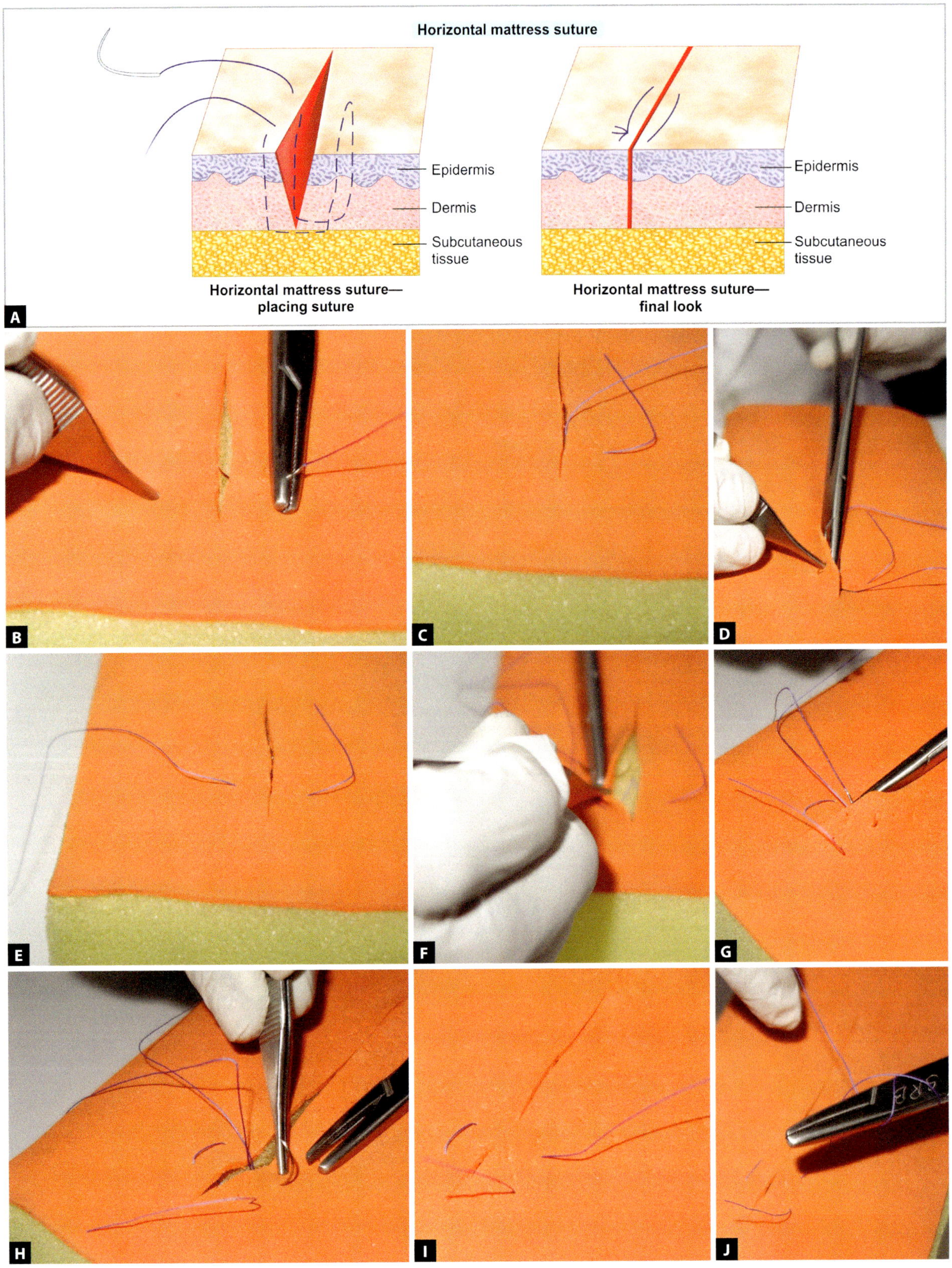

**Figs. 20A to J**

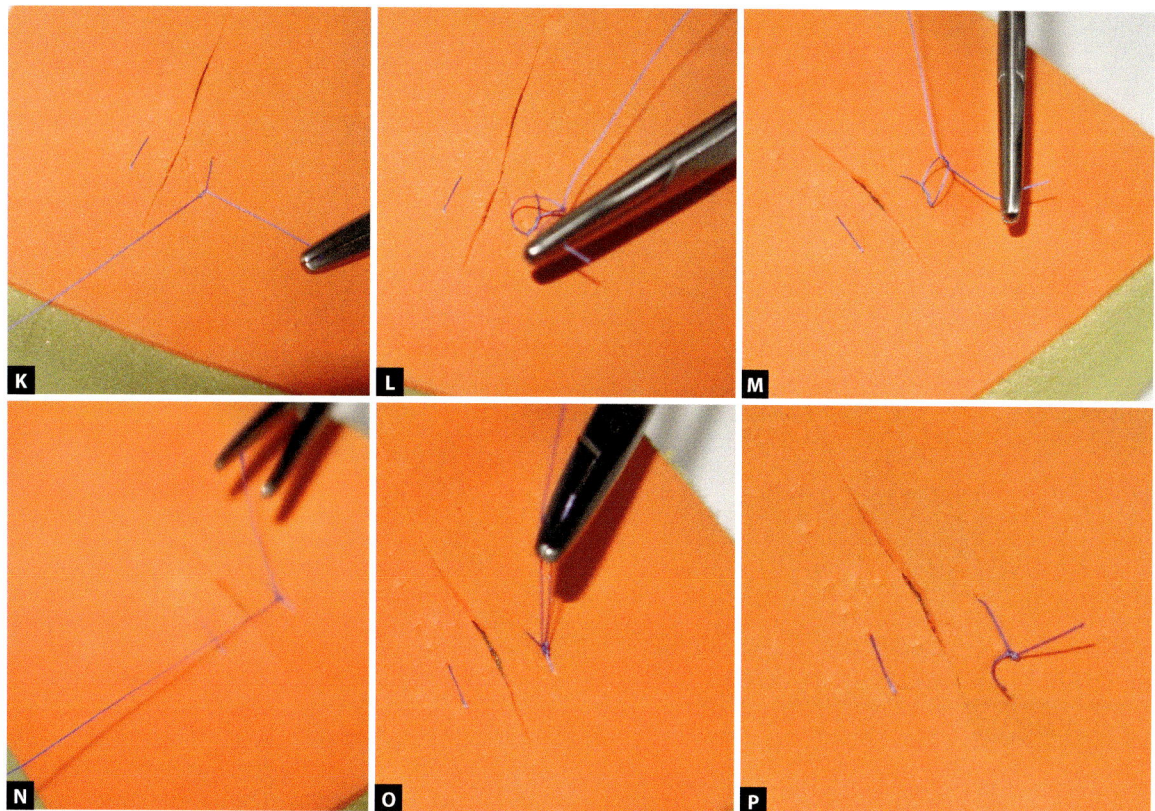

**Figs. 20K to P**

**Figs. 20A to P:** Horizontal mattress suture.

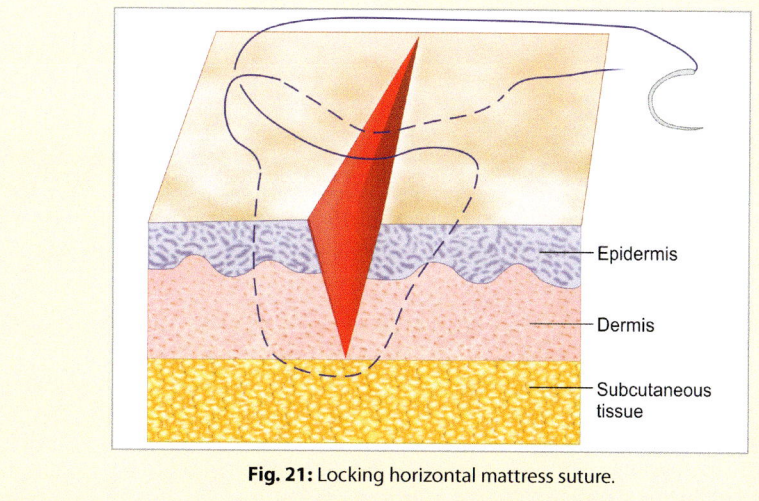

**Fig. 21:** Locking horizontal mattress suture.

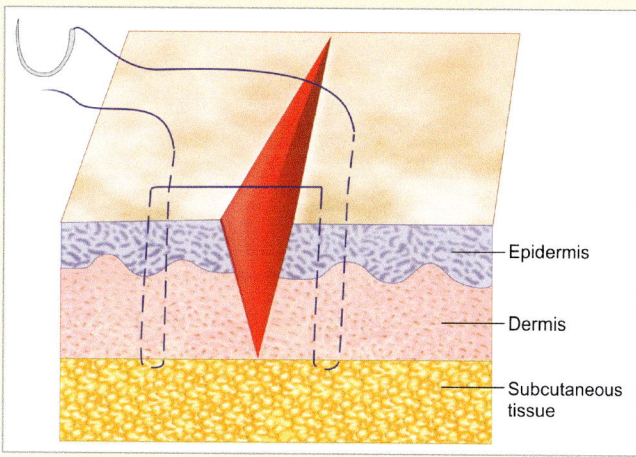

**Fig. 22:** Inverting horizontal mattress suture.

**64** SRB's Atlas of Tissue Approximation with Suturing and Knotting

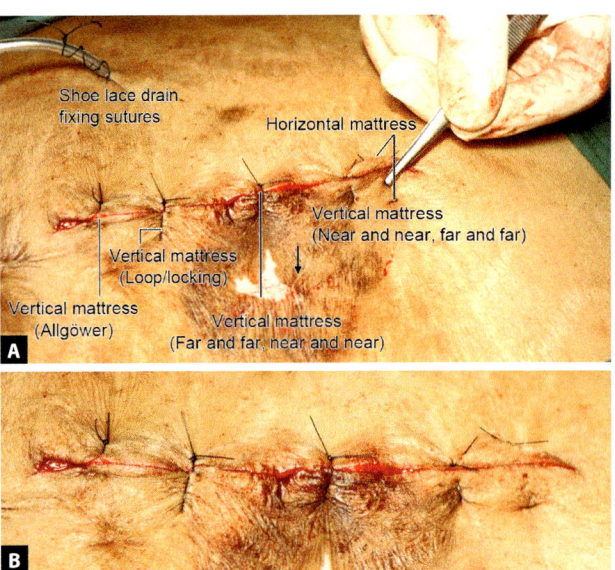

**Figs. 23A and B:** Different types of sutures—vertical and horizontal mattress types.

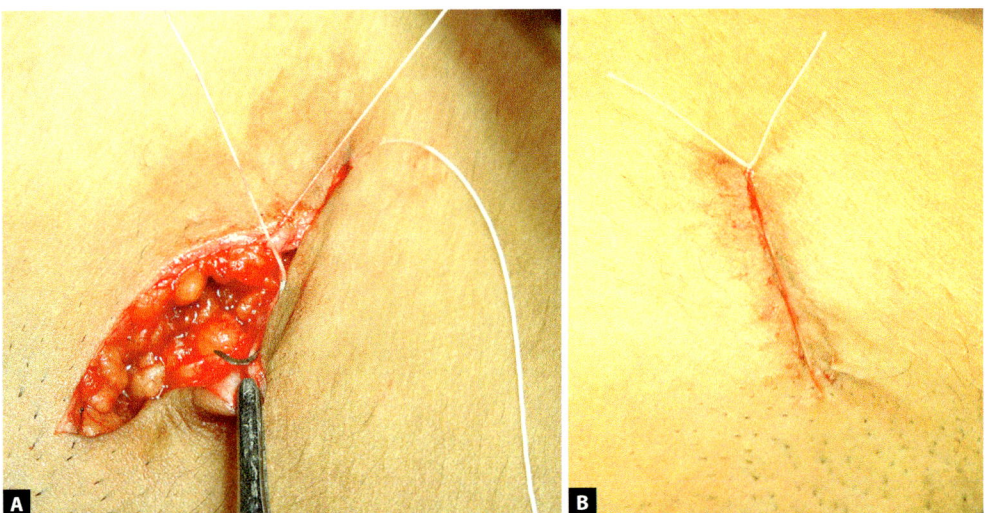

**Figs. 24A and B:** Technique of subcuticular suture placing.

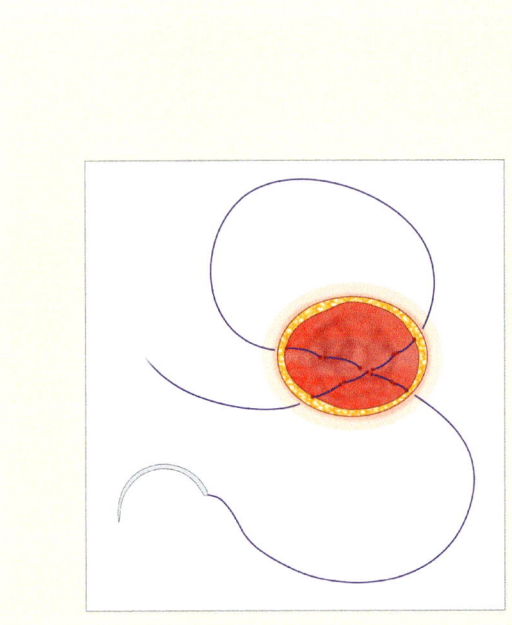

**Fig. 25:** Figure of eight suture.

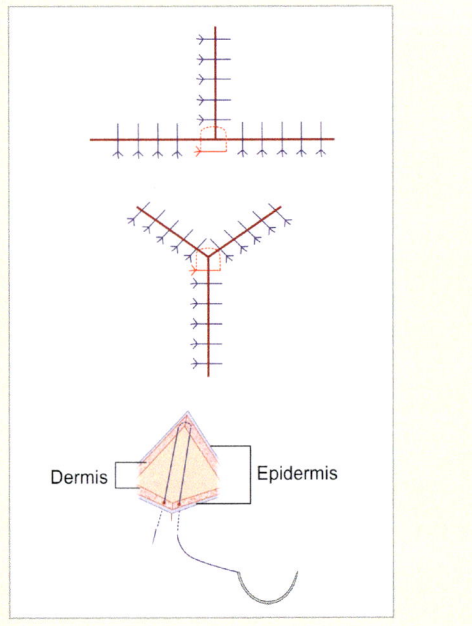

**Fig. 26:** Three-point suturing is used in apposing junction of the triangular flaps.

wound edge. Advantage is—it is easier to place. It is stronger and holds well. It is used in small wound. Figure of eight is similar one used in depth as well as surface on the tissue surface mainly to control bleeding **(Fig. 28)**.

### Quilled Suture

It is done in abdominal wall and other areas where strong tension is needed to appose the wound edges and to prevent possible chance of wound dehiscence. Tubes are placed on either sides of the wound edge. Vertical mattress sutures are placed wherein tubes are made to stay within the loops of the mattress sutures **(Fig. 29)**.

### Retention Sutures (Tension Sutures)

It is even though practiced in many centers, ideally, it should be avoided. It is used during closure of laparotomies done for acute conditions such as peritonitis, intestinal obstruction wherein patient's general condition is not good; layer-by-layer closure may cause acute wound failure with burst abdomen; when quick closure is a need of the day. Its use is getting replaced by *Smead-Jones* sutures or interrupted single layer deeper sutures. Retention sutures are taken as full thickness sutures placed 3–5 cm away from the wound. Large curved cutting needle is used. Number 0 or 1 monofilament suture material-like polyethylene is used. First bite is taken away from the wound from skin to peritoneum into the peritoneal cavity; needle is then brought back 3–5 cm away from the opposite edge of the wound; suture material is passed through a supportive sterile tube (cut-drip set tube) of 2–3 cm length; near the edge of the skin of the existing side needle and suture material is passed; similar bite is taken on the same side of skin edge; suture is passed through one more sterile tube of 2–3 cm size and is kept ready for knotting after completion of placing all sutures. Each suture is placed with a gap of 1.5–2 cm. Knotting is started from one corner; but if closure is difficult then central knot is put first. While knotting in deeper plane, bowel, and omentum should be guarded with finger or by placing mop or using a special curved bow-like instrument (*Sergeant instrument*) so as to prevent entangling or injuring these structures. Sutures are cut once all knots are tied on one side of the wound. Skin may be apposed using separate sutures.

*In vertical mattress retention sutures*, tubes cross the wound. *In horizontal mattress retention sutures*, bites are taken like a square and sterile tubes are placed parallel to the wound (not crossing). In this, type number of sutures needed is

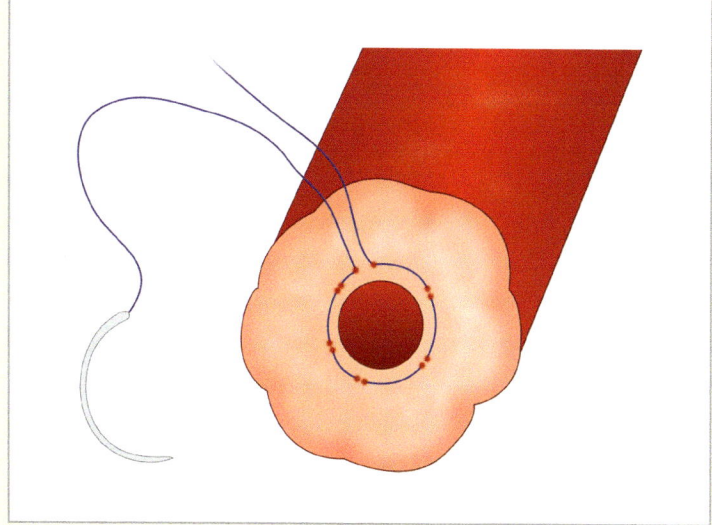

**Fig. 27:** Purse-string suture.

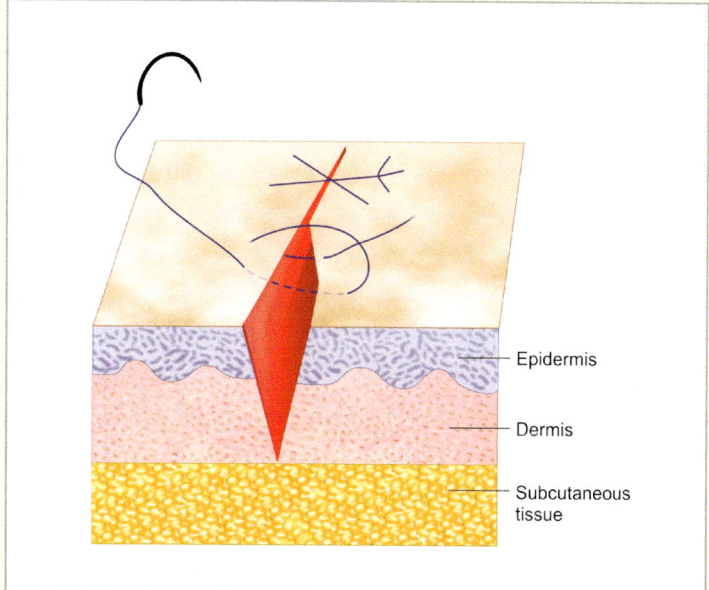

**Fig. 28:** Interrupted cruciate suture.

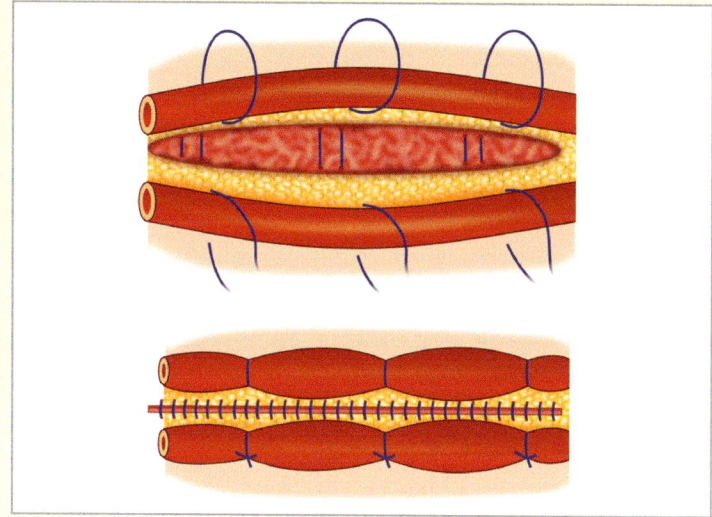

**Fig. 29:** Quilled suture.

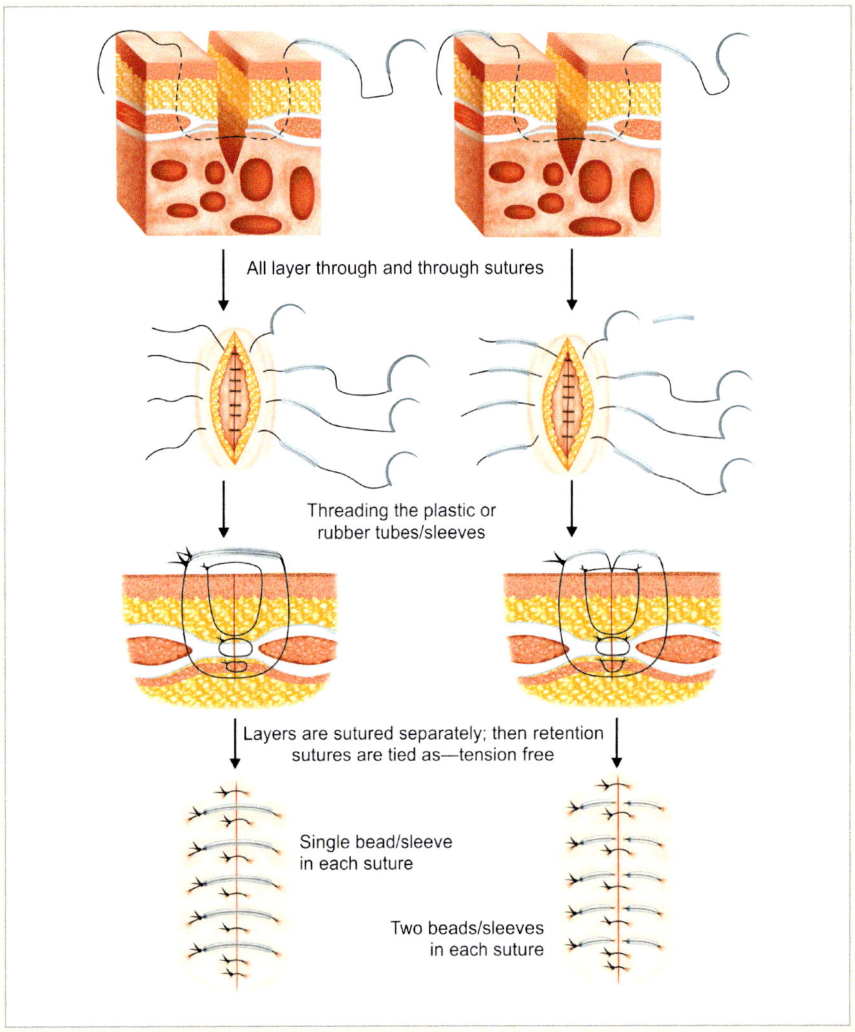

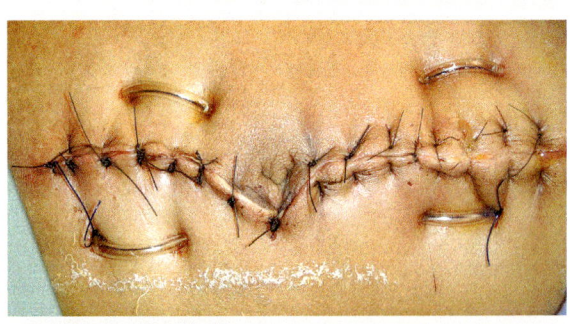

**Fig. 30:** Retention sutures.

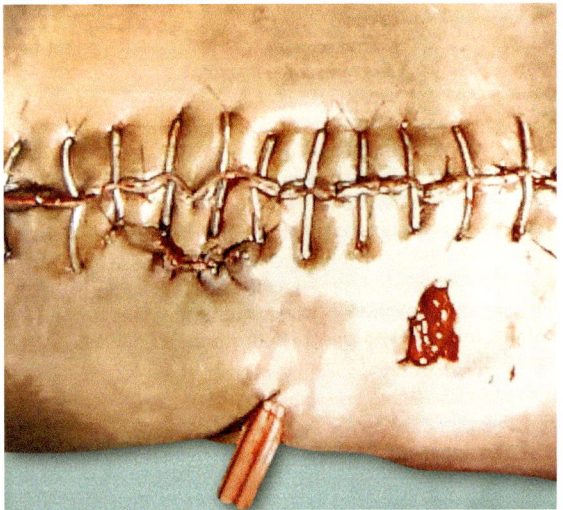

**Fig. 31:** Vertical mattress retention sutures. It is full thickness single layer suture.

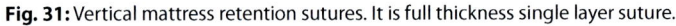

**Fig. 32:** Horizontal mattress suture.

less than vertical type. Distinct advantages of horizontal mattress retention suture type are not clear but it is said that it is stronger than vertical mattress retention suture. But chances of bowel or omentum getting trapped are higher in this **(Figs. 30 to 32)**.

*Modified Smead-Jones closure:* It is interrupted specialized suture used in the closure of abdomen as single layer excluding the skin. Linea alba is held with Allis' forceps. *Number one* polyamide or PDS suture material is used. First bite on one side taken 3 cm away (width) from the margin from outside to inside; it is then passed through the corresponding opposite edge with 3 cm width from inside to outside; later again one small loop of 5 mm width from the edges of each side of the wound from first bite site to second bite site is taken; suture is knotted on the free edge of the first bite side. Full thickness bite holds the suture and maintains the tension in the wound. Smaller loop keeps the linea alba in apposed place. Large curved *Ferguson needle* is better to place these sutures. Each suture is placed at 2 cm interval. Instead of retention sutures, modified Smead–Jones method is used during closure after laparotomy in acute abdominal conditions. Here also, it is better to place all sutures under proper vision and knotting is done at the end. At least, four knots should be placed. Excessive tension should be avoided. In upper abdomen, peritoneum need not be included in the bite; but in lower abdomen as linea alba is indistinct, peritoneum is included in this **(Fig. 33)**.

*LE Hughes double near and far suture:* It is similar with same indications as Smead–Jones, with double near and far sutures placed to have a strong loop with knot on one side **(Fig. 34)**.

*Single layer seromucosal suture of bowel:* It is now well-practiced method of suturing of the bowel. Interrupted seromucosal sutures using 3-0/2-0 Vicryl or PDS takes up well. Nonabsorbable silk or linen also can be used. These nonabsorbable sutures are good old suture materials which are even now accepted well. Only drawback presumed is formation of suture granuloma at the anastomotic site **(Fig. 35)**.

*Gambee single layer full thickness (all layers) sutures:* It is done using Vicryl and is also used in bowel anastomosis. It can also be used as continuous sutures especially during gastrojejunostomy. *Continuous suturing* is quicker; alternate bites should be locked to prevent purse-string effect; anterior layer is closed with inverting sutures. *Interrupted suture* is more stable and stronger with less chances of anastomotic disruption. It also maintains the blood supply better than continuous sutures. Width of suture bite taken should be less over mucosal part than seromuscular part. Bites are taken 3 mm from the cut edge of the serosa; each bite is taken in a 5-mm gap **(Fig. 36)**.

### Lembert Suture

It is the most commonly used seromuscular suture. Silk 3-0 or Vicryl 3-0 is used. Deep seromuscular suture including submucosal layer is taken at a point 5 mm from the cut edge of the serosa; this bite emerges at same line closure at 2 mm from the cut edge of serosa; bite is taken on the opposite part of the bowel at 2 mm from the serosal cut edge as seromuscular which emerges at 5 mm point away in the same longitudinal line and knot is placed. It can be used as continuous suture also **(Fig. 37)**.

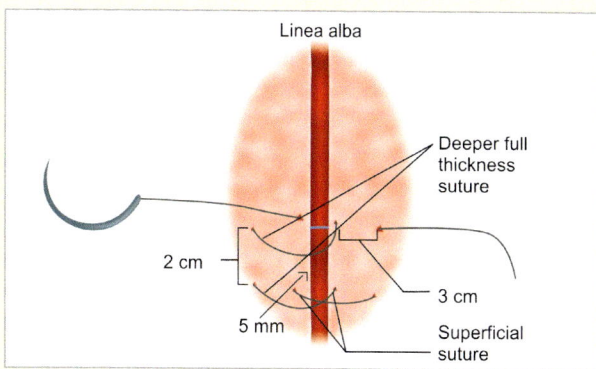

**Fig. 33:** Modified Smead–Jones sutures. These sutures are better than placing retention sutures.

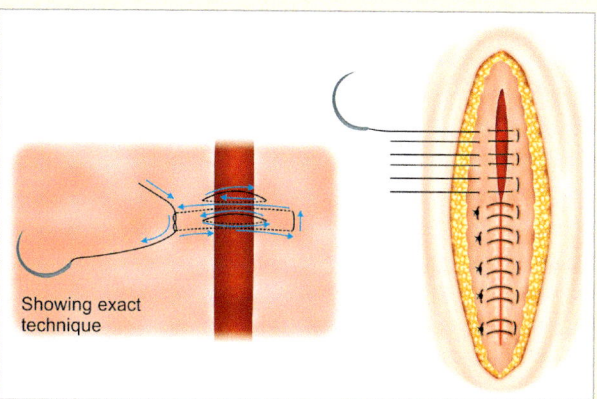

**Fig. 34:** LE Hughes double near and far suture.

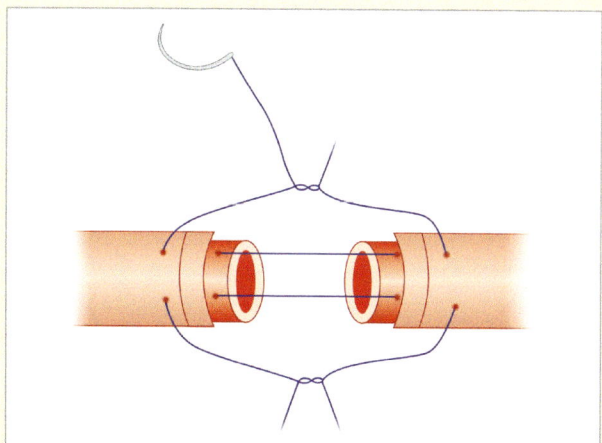

**Fig. 35:** Single layer seromucosal layer suturing of the bowel.

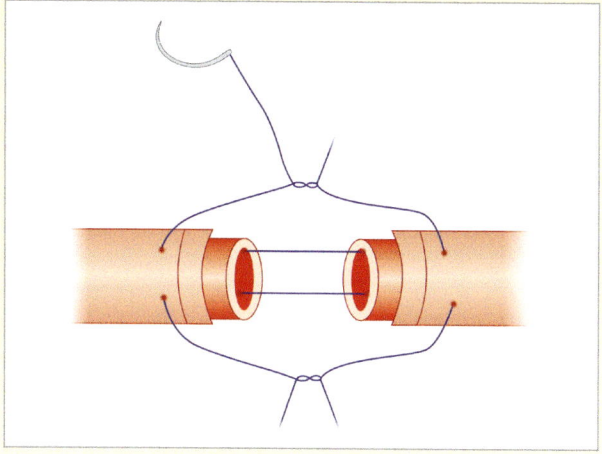

**Fig. 36:** Gambee suture.

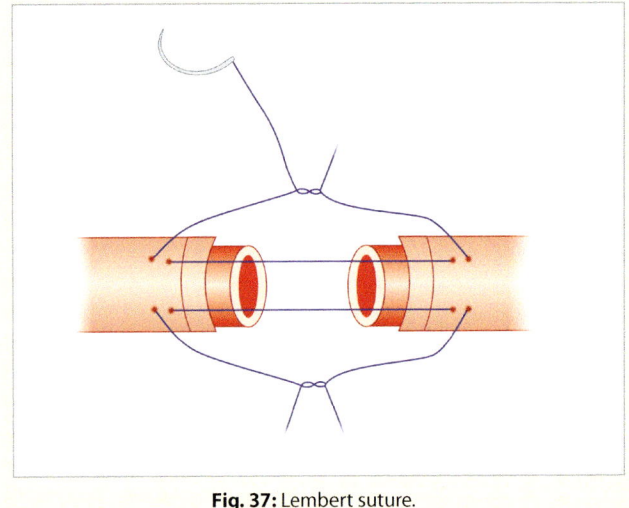

Fig. 37: Lembert suture.     Fig. 38: Cushing suture.

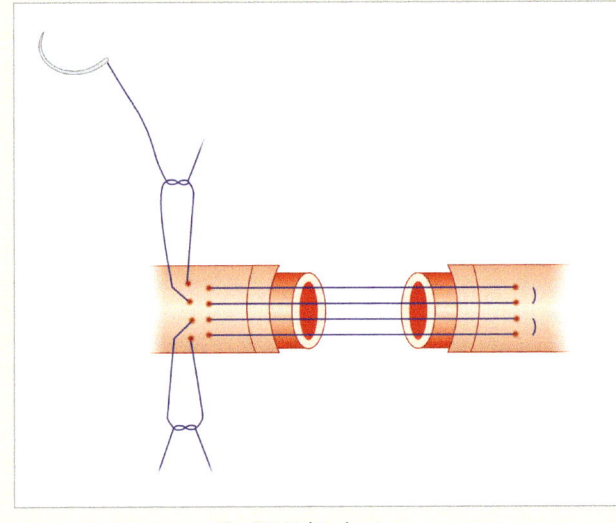 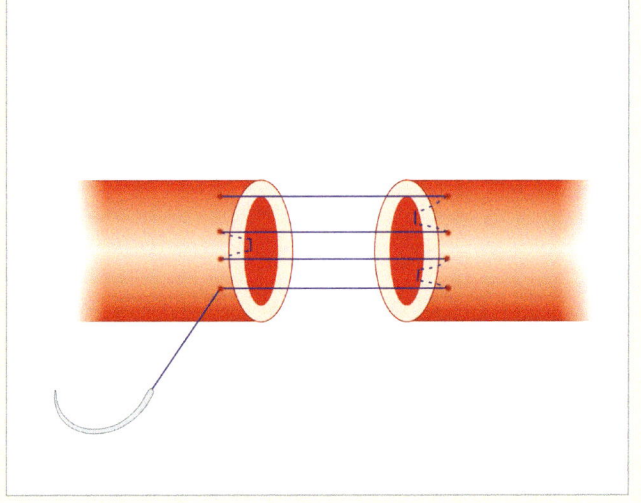

Fig. 39: Halsted suture.     Fig. 40: Connell suture for bowel anastomosis.

### Cushing Suture

It is similar to Lembert suture wherein seromuscular bites are taken parallel to the cut edge of the serosa (at 2 mm from the cut edge). Thickness of tissue taken is 5 mm. Both interrupted and continuous sutures can be taken **(Fig. 38)**.

### Halsted Suture

It is actually seromuscular horizontal mattress suture. Care must be taken to avoid excessive tension over the suture line as this may lead into ischemia of the anastomotic site **(Fig. 39)**.

### Connell Suture

Here suture material passes through all the layers of the intestine from serosa to mucosa; again brought out through all layers of the intestine on the same side from mucosa to serosa; passed over opposite segment of the bowel; passing from serosa to lumen/mucosa and from mucosa to outside towards serosa; again coming towards the same side to repeat the technique. It is very good technique to invert the mucosal part of the anterior layer. It is commonly used in double layer anastomosis but can be used in single layer anastomosis. Connell suture apposes well; achieves good mucosal inversion. But it is *not adequately hemostatic* and so bleeders on the cut edge of the bowel should be ligated or cauterized individually **(Fig. 40)**.

# CHAPTER 7: Laparoscopic Suturing and Knotting

> "The good physician treats the disease; the great physician treats the patient who has the disease."
> —Sir William Osler
>
> "Peeping Toms" are condemned; but "peeping surgeons" are hailed.
> —Quote
>
> "A knot, irrespective of its nature, has to be configured correctly or else it is hopelessly wrong."
> —Dictum of Ashley

## INTRODUCTION

Laparoscopic suturing and knot tying are a challenging task in laparoscopic surgery.

*Problems with laparoscopic suturing are*—lack of tissue perception, depth, limitation of movement of the instruments, difficulty in suturing and knotting inside, restricted space of working, and need for high-skill level by the laparoscopic surgeon. It can be intracorporeal and extracorporeal knots. Both suturing and knot tying are individual challenges. Extracorporeal is easier as knot is made outside and passed through the port and reducer to slip the knot at required site. Different extracorporeal knots are practiced. There is no tactile feel and depth perception in laparoscopic suturing. There is minimal peripheral vision in laparoscopic surgery causing loss of workspace for efficient navigation of instruments. Grasping efficiency and transfer of force from handle to tip in laparoscopic instrument is 1 : 3 as compared to open surgery instruments, where grasping force transfer is 3 : 1 ratio creating surgeon to use six times compulsorily more force. Freedom of movement in laparoscopic instrument is only 4°, limiting the dexterity. Handling suture material, needle positioning, and maneuverability; getting proper bites; withdrawing the needle from the wound edge; and knotting—all are challenging part of the laparoscopic suturing and knotting. Laparoscopic view and continuous clarity image getting are also often a challenge. Ergonomics, triangulation, stance, concentration, motivation, discipline, dexterity, coordination, repetitive learning, and practice are essential to learn this art. Hand–eye coordination and visual perception and concentration are important. In open surgery, there is high degree of freedom and one can work in line with visual axis. There is three-dimensional direct vision with direct tactile feel. In laparoscopy, there is two-dimensional vision without tactile feel and depth perception. Manipulation angle should be 45–75° with equal azimuth angles to have optimum performance in dissection and mainly suturing and knotting (best angle is 60°); if more, it gives extra workload to deltoid and trapezius muscles; if less, it causes poor performance. When optical trocar is placed as one of the lateral port trocar, it is called as *sectorization*. Optical trocar should be placed in the central port to have *triangulation which is natural position for the surgeon* **(Figs. 1A and B)**. Sectorization is done only if need arises like in laparoscopic appendicectomy **(Fig. 2)**.

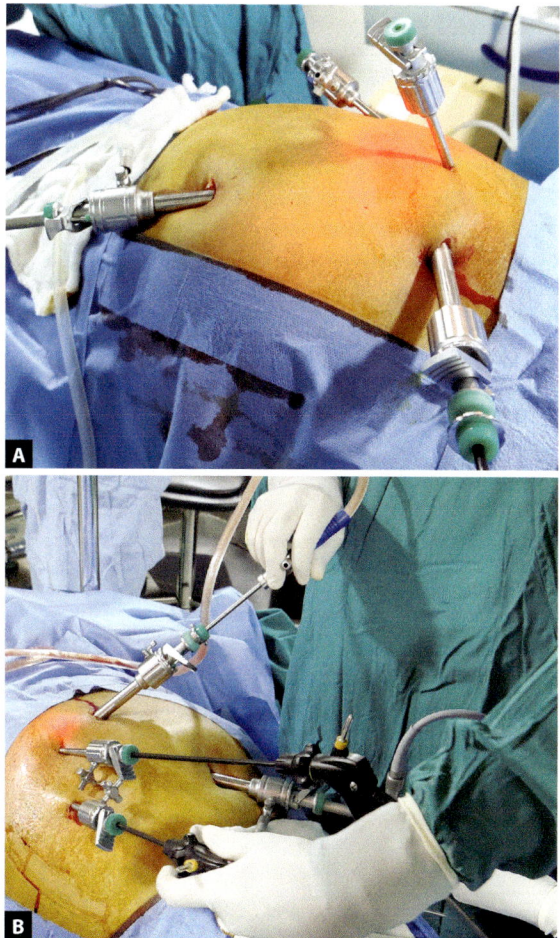

**Figs. 1A and B:** Natural position for the surgeon with "triangulation" of working ports on both sides of the central camera.

*Note:* Any individual performs a skill better and with more caution whenever he has the knowledge that he is under observation and assessment—*Hawthorne effect*. This holds very good to laparoscopic surgery.

*Prerequisites for laparoscopic suturing:*
- Perfect health—mentally and physically
- Hand—eye coordination
- Visual perception, ability to concentrate, dedication, and determination
- Precision, proper camera operator
- Learning curve, repetitive training, motivation, discipline, and willpower
- Proper instruments and their usage
- Triangulation of two working instruments is important.

## TYPES OF LAPAROSCOPIC SUTURING AND KNOTTING

Two types are used in laparoscopic suturing and knotting (mainly knotting)—*extracorporeal and intracorporeal types*. Even though extracorporeal looks easier than intracorporeal, both types need concentration, learning, and application while configuring them. Both need proper knowledge of execution with perfect principles.

### Extracorporeal Knotting

It is commonly advocated in laparoscopy, as it is convenient, safe, and effective. Long, 90 cm, suture is used; needle with suture may be passed through tissue inside under laparoscopic vision and brought out through the 5-mm/10-mm port. Similarly, ligature also can be looped around the specific structure and ends of the suture are brought out for knotting. After placing extracorporeal knotting, it is pushed to the required site through a *knot pusher* (**Fig. 3**). Additional knots similarly can be placed. Knot is tied and drawn externally and then slipped down into the target site with knot pusher and when traction is given to the stranding end of the suture material, which extends long outside the port instrument. *Throw/knot pusher* may be plastic single use or metallic multiple use. These instruments push slip knots already created into the target tissue. Metallic reusable knot pusher has got groove/slit/fork at the tip to place the knot and suture.

It is very useful in ligating the vessels greater than 4 mm, as it is more secure and holds tight. It is used in ligating tubular structures like appendix, gallbladder (after retrograde dissection); in areas where there is limited space for intracorporeal maneuver. Length of the suture material should be long enough, so that its stranding end adequately comes out of the port so as to avail the proper tightening of the knot through knot pusher. Endoloops are disposable preformed knot suture material

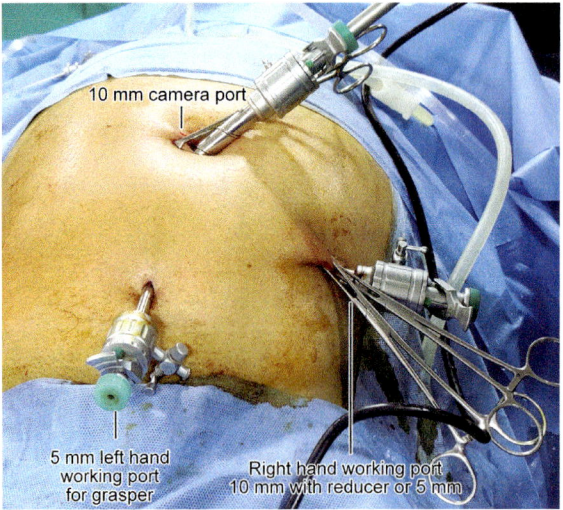

**Fig. 2:** Sectorization—port position is used in laparoscopic appendicectomy; there is no proper triangulation here as per principle. Here, working instrument ports are on one side of the laparoscope. This is "offset" position.

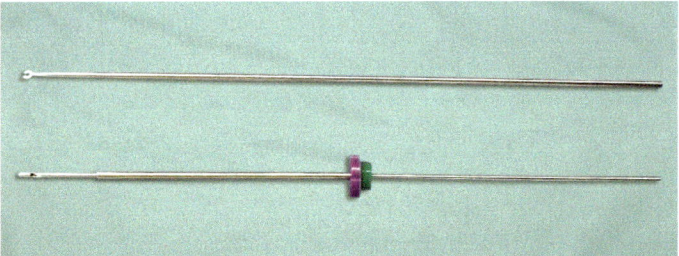

**Fig. 3:** Knot pusher for guiding and placing extracorporeal knots in laparoscopic surgery.

with a one-time pusher of the knot (**Figs. 4 and 5**). 2-0 or 1-0 suture materials are ideal. Catgut slips well as well as polyglactin 910 (Vicryl). Braided suture slips well and will not get loosened by slip back unlike monofilament sutures. Catgut shows high resistance for *reverse slipping*. Silk and Vicryl are also can be used. Different knot pushers are available—*open loop knot pusher* and *push rod type*. Melzer's knot pusher has got outer cutting sleeve, which when activated cuts the ligature after the knot has been locked and tightened.

When extracorporeal knot is done and is pushed, it needs double length of the suture material—around 90–150-cm length suture material. Free end of the suture is passed into the 5-mm port or through 5-mm reducer across the 10-mm port using a laparoscopic needle holder (presentation), insertion into the peritoneal cavity, looping of the tissue or tubular structure (example cystic duct), exteriorization of the open loop, external knotting, slipping the knot to the target site, and locking and tightening the knot. While presenting the suture, it should be held by the tip of the needle holder rather than proximally.

*Different types of extracorporeal knots are:*
- Roeder's knot (By Roeder—used for tonsillectomy in 1918): Semm used this in laparoscopy. Catgut is commonly used. Silk and 2-0 Vicryl also can be used. Initial half knot (single loop) → 3½ turns over the loop → second half knot → pushing toward first loop → tightening creates good Roeder's knot, which can be slid over the suture material easily → pushed after loop is passed around the structure like base of appendix using knot pusher (**Figs. 6 and 7**).
- *Melzer's knot (Melzer, Germany, 1991):* It is modification of Roeder's knot (**Fig. 8**). Here double initial half knot (double loop) → 3½ turn over the limbs of the loop → double second half knot → staking of turns and pushing to tighten the knot → ready for use with a loop. It is used with PDS and is *stronger* than Roeder's knot.
- *Tayside knot:* Initial half knot → 4½ turn loop on standing part → tail is passed through first loop → tail is again passed through the first loop → tail is pulled to tighten the knot and ready for use. It is modified Fisherman's utility knot (Scotland) (**Fig. 9**).
- *Duncan slip knot:* Half hitch is added to the loop after 3½ turn (**Fig. 10**).
- *Texas Endosurgery Institute Knot (TEI Knot):* It is useful for many suture materials like PDS but it is difficult to do and several methods are present.

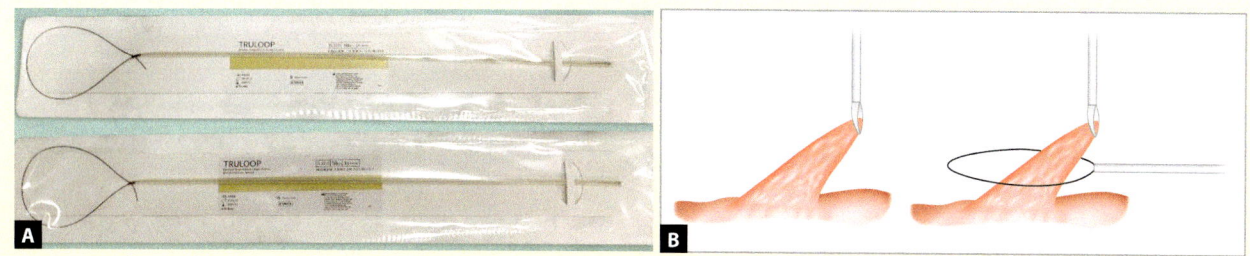

**Figs. 4A and B:** Endoloop used in ligating tubular structures. It is mainly used in laparoscopic appendicectomy. Minimum two ligatures should be placed proximally for safe ligation. It may be pretied endoloop (chromic catgut) or endoloop is made using Roeder's knot with Vicryl. Pretied plastic endoloop has got push rod, which after introducing into the abdominal cavity and looping around the target tissue proximally is broken to allow the distal part of pushrod to push the knot into the tissue securely.

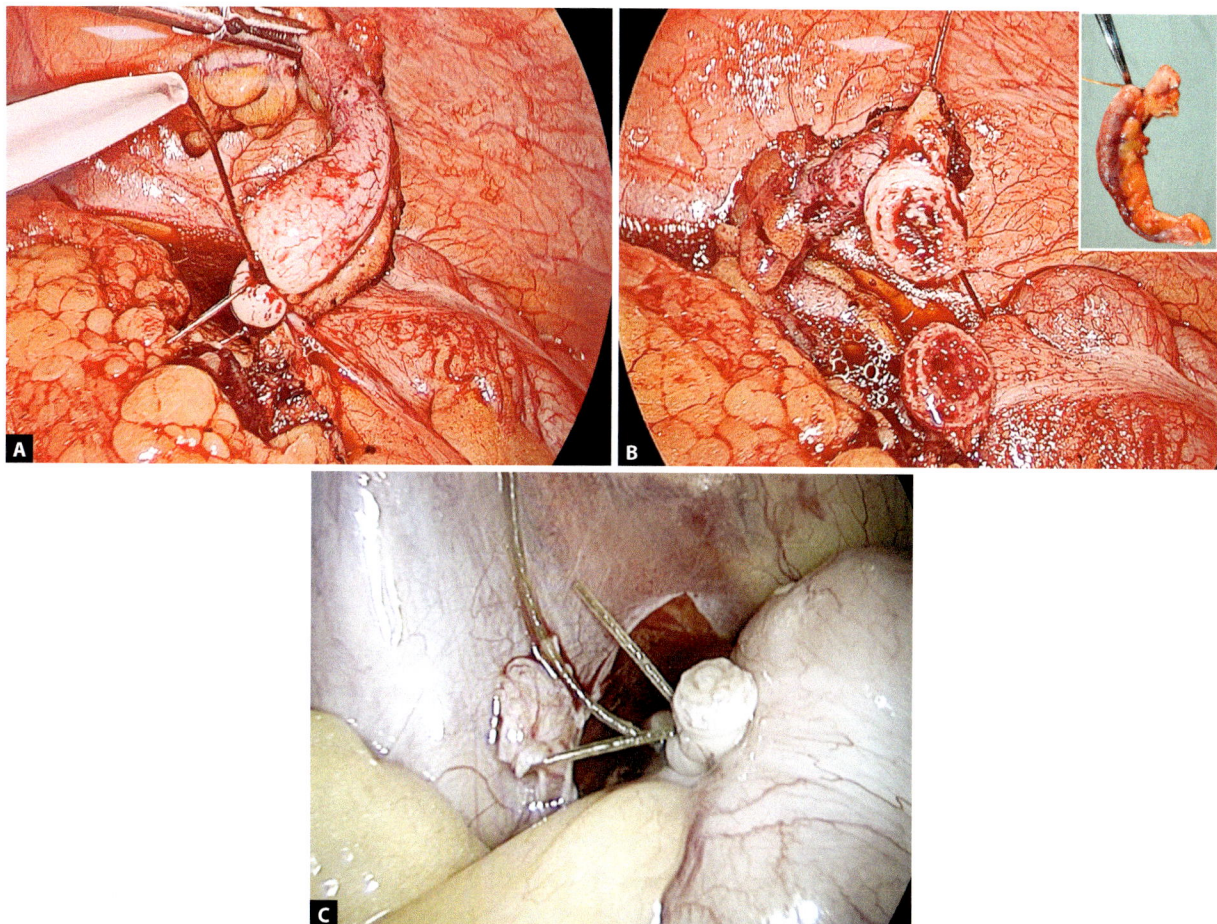

**Figs. 5A to C:** Laparoscopic appendicectomy endoloop in position.

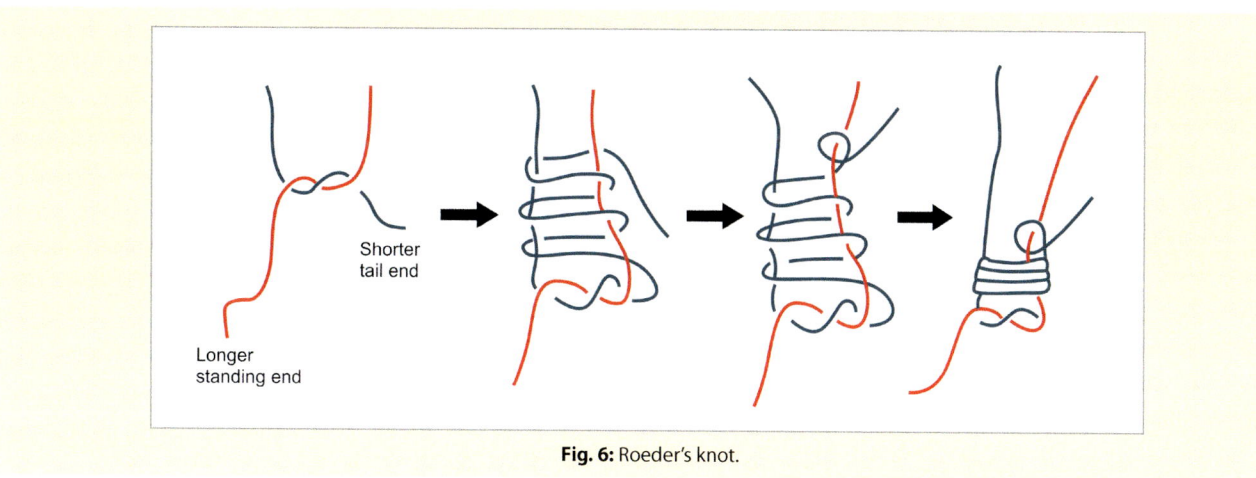

**Fig. 6:** Roeder's knot.

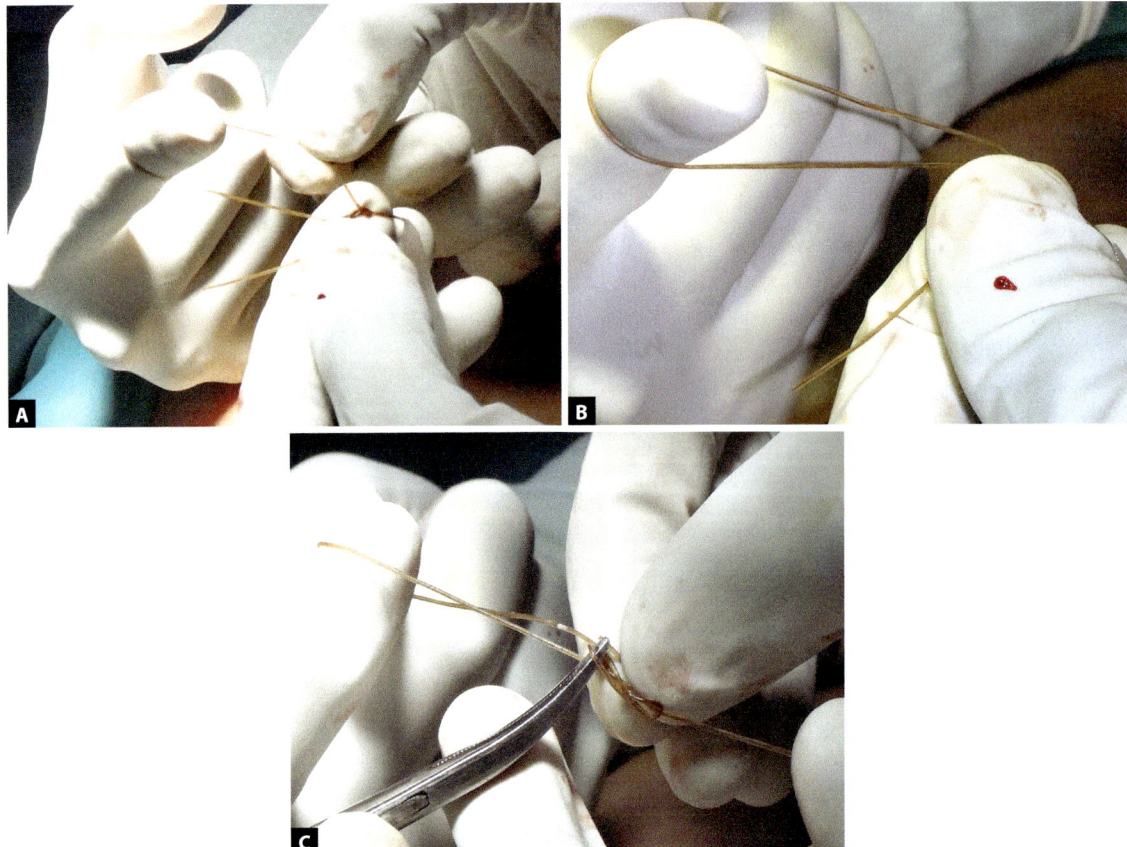

**Figs. 7A to C:** Technique of creating Roeder's knot.

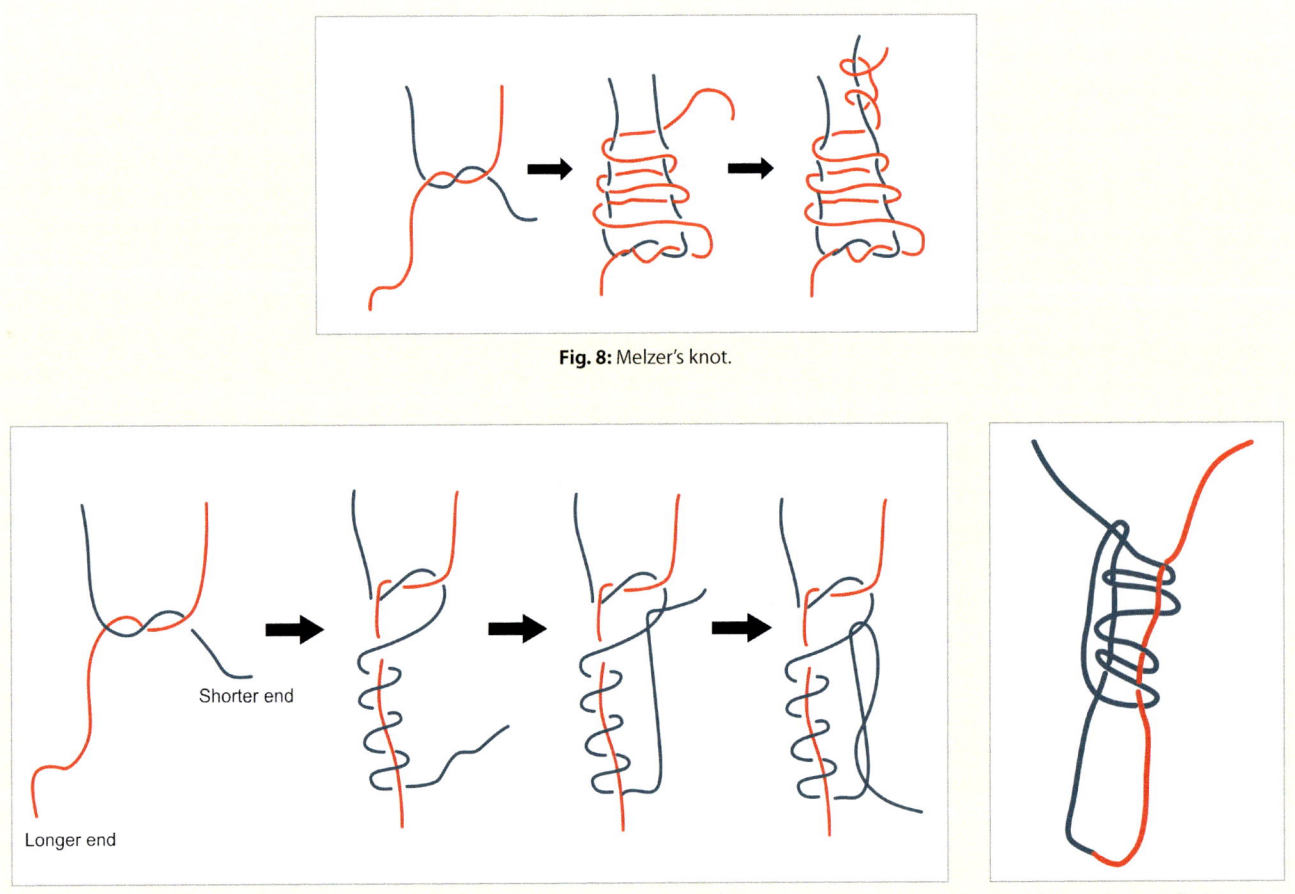

**Fig. 8:** Melzer's knot.

**Fig. 9:** Tayside knot.

**Fig. 10:** Duncan slip knot.

*Note: Other extracorporeal knots are—blood knots, modified blood knots, cross square knots, and eye hook knots. Readers can refer specialized books for the same, as they are beyond the scope of this book and are not commonly used.*

*Preformed slip knots—endoloops:* These are prelooped sutures which are commonly used in appendicectomy, cholecystectomy, or ligating blood vessels. Chromic catgut is the material commonly used here. It is introduced and placed using 5-mm endoloop pusher. Disposable pushers with preknotted endoloops are available. Metal knot pusher is not disposable (reusable) with a Roeder's knot.

*Extracorporeal knots:* These are used in ligating base of the appendix, bleeding vessels of 3-mm size, ligation of the cystic duct in difficult retrograde cholecystectomy, pedicle ligation, and ligation of indirect hernia sac.

*In laparoscopic appendicectomy, for example,* grasper (Maryland also can be used) is passed through left hand instrument; endoloop (Roeder's knot) is passed through the right-hand trocar (10 mm with reducer or 5 mm); appendix is held using left-hand instrument; it is released to allow loop to pass through the appendix and manipulated to reach the proper base of the appendix; again, appendix is held distally firmly with grasper and is given to assistant/scrub nurse to hold it raised position firmly; right-hand trocar with loop and knot pusher should be in line and there should not be any gap between the knot and the instrument to have proper sliding of the knot toward the target site. Often tip of the knot pusher is positioned over the base/target site firmly and knot is pushed towards it so that knot slipping towards the target point is made easier. Once knot is firmly tightened, knot pusher is released and kept lax away from the base of the appendix; through left-hand port, grasper is replaced with scissor to cut the suture material. One more suture ligation just proximally and another still proximally are placed. Appendix is the cut using right-hand instrument using curved tissue scissor **(Figs. 11 and 12)**.

## Intracorporeal Suturing and Knotting

It is technically demanding one. Fine needle with suture is used. *Ski needle* with rounded curved tip and triangular straight shaft is also often used. Needle is held at triangular shaft, so that needle will not swivel. *Dundee "Ski" needle* **(Fig. 13)** with flattened proximal cross-section instead of triangular makes improved locking and fixation of needle into needle holder without much difficulty, which makes positioning of the needle easier. Standard curved needles are also commonly used but with swiveling problem. Polyfilament, colored (black or fluorescent white), and 3-0 suture materials are ideal. Polyfilament material holds well with easy knotting ability.

Excellent needle holder is an asset for intracorporeal knotting. Semm, Wolf, Ethicon, Cook, MBG are different needle holders available. Szabo and Berci needle holder gives 360° rotation with precise maneuvering. *Self-righting needle holder* with a notch inside allowing self-positioning of the needle is also available. *Coaxial needle holder and pistol needle holders* are available. *Self-righting needle holder* is also available wherein needle gets automatically adjusted in curved position making needle placement easier **(Figs. 14 to 16)**.

Needle with suture material is placed inside the peritoneal cavity through: (1) 5-mm reducer across 10-mm port; (2) Direct percutaneous (only straight needle or curved needle in thin patients and

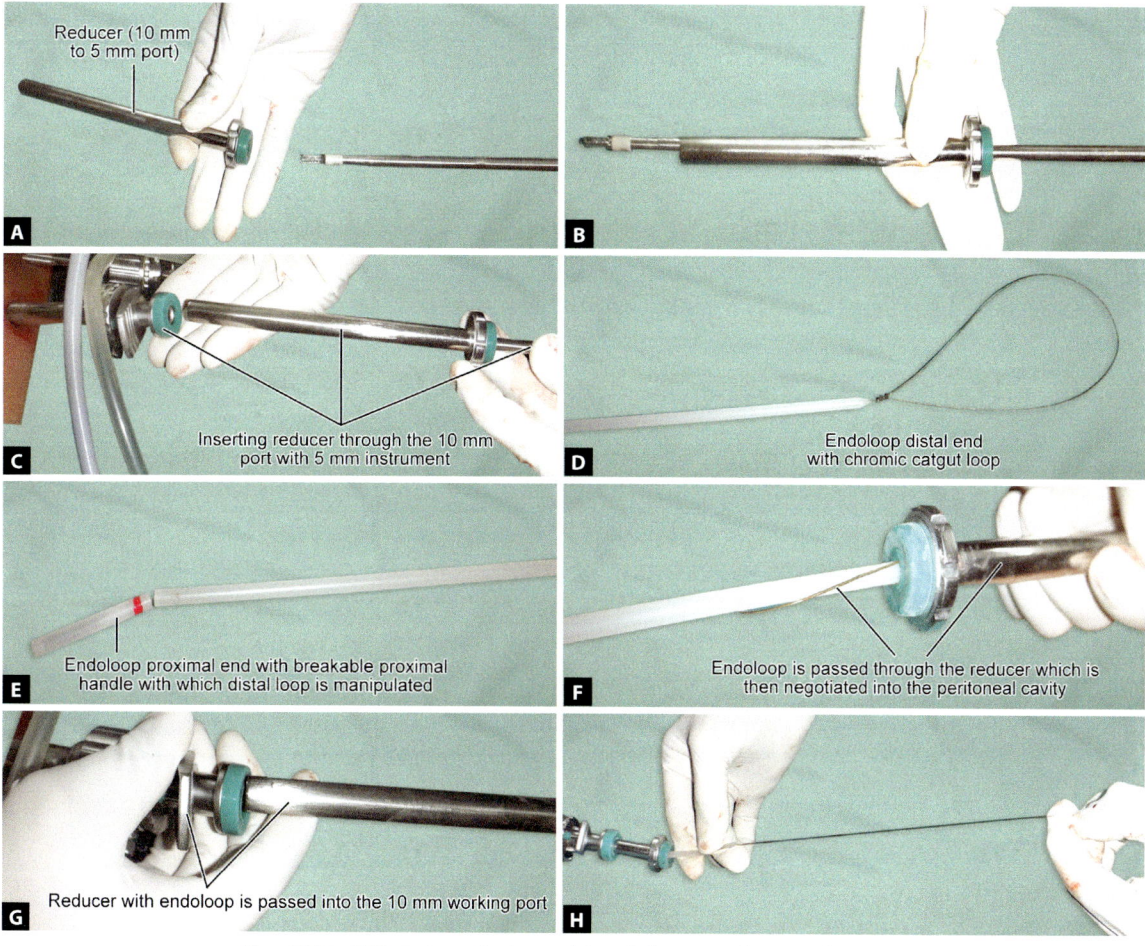

**Figs. 11A to H:** Technique of using endoloop in laparoscopic appendicectomy.

children); (3) *Reich method* through 5-mm port (5-mm port is removed gently, needle with 5-mm needle holder is directly pushed along the track of the removed port into the peritoneal cavity under laparoscope guidance and 5-mm port is again slid into the abdominal cavity across needle holder); and (4) Through 10-mm port directly. Needle entangling in the tissues, needle cutting, separation of the suture material from the needle, and injury to the vital organs are the problems, which may occur while introducing the needle.

Entrance bite and exit bite in the tissue should be taken separately. Knot is formed

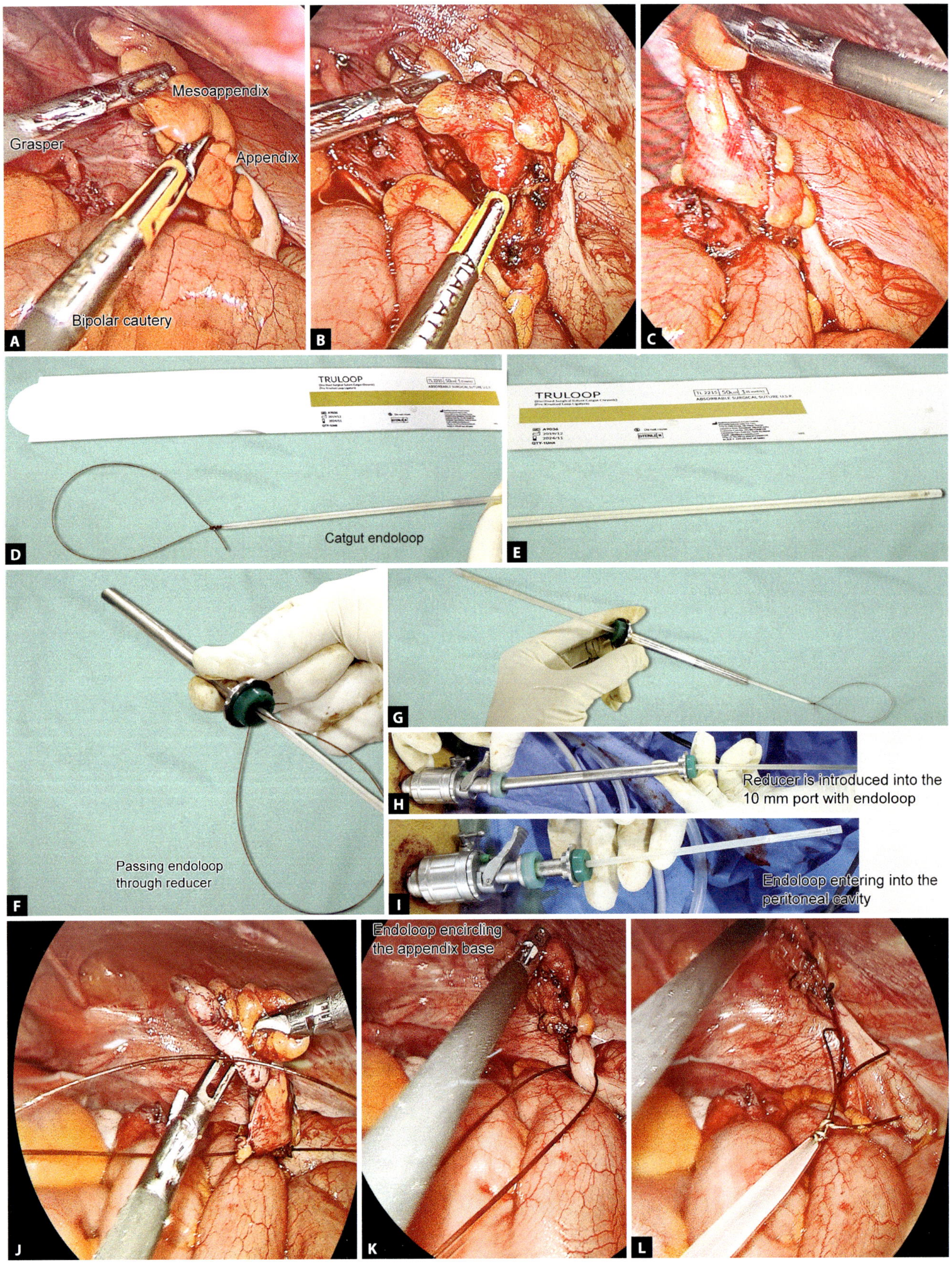

Figs. 12A to L

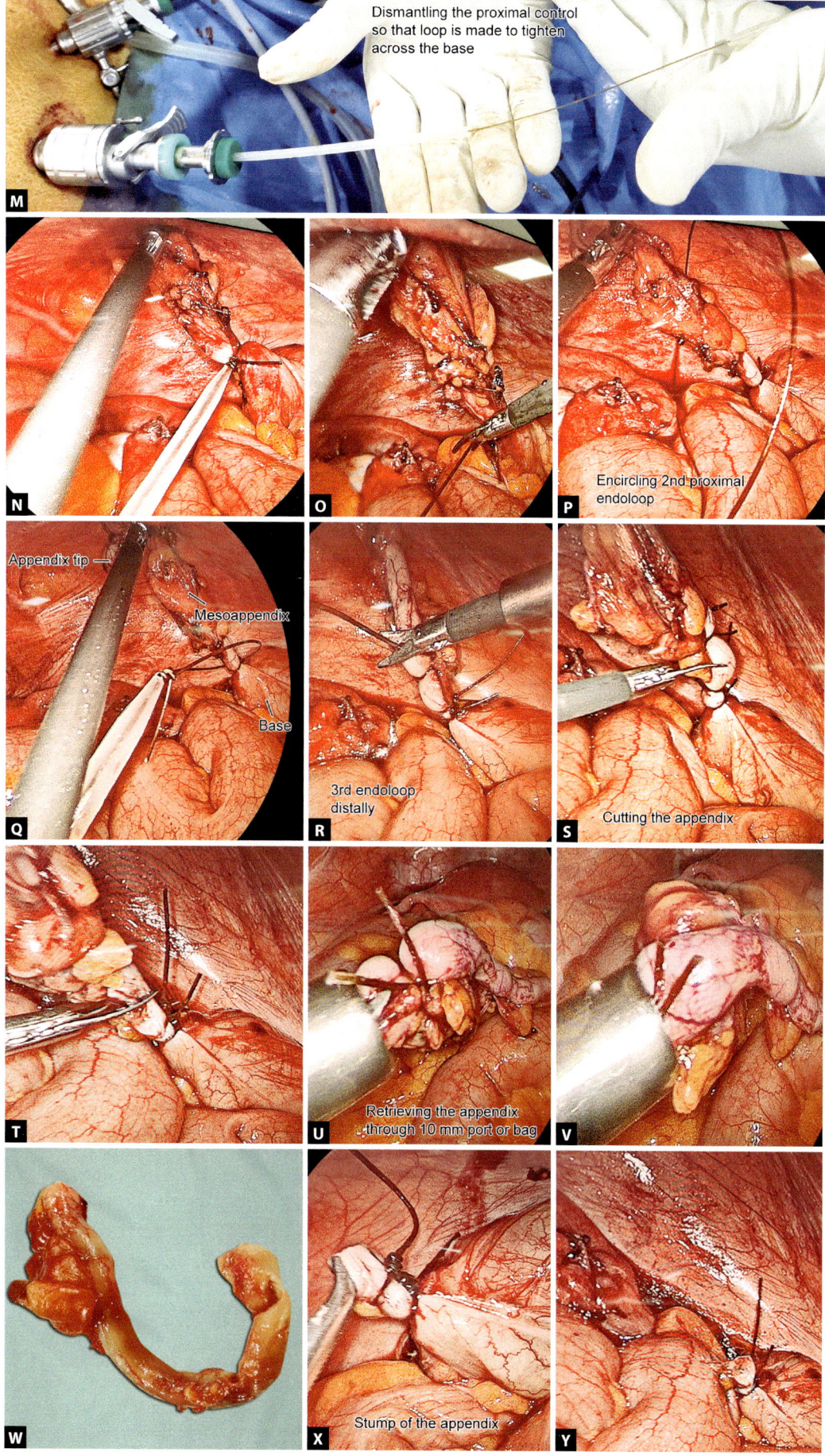

**Figs. 12M to Y**

**Figs. 12A to Y:** Laparoscopic appendicectomy using endoloop.

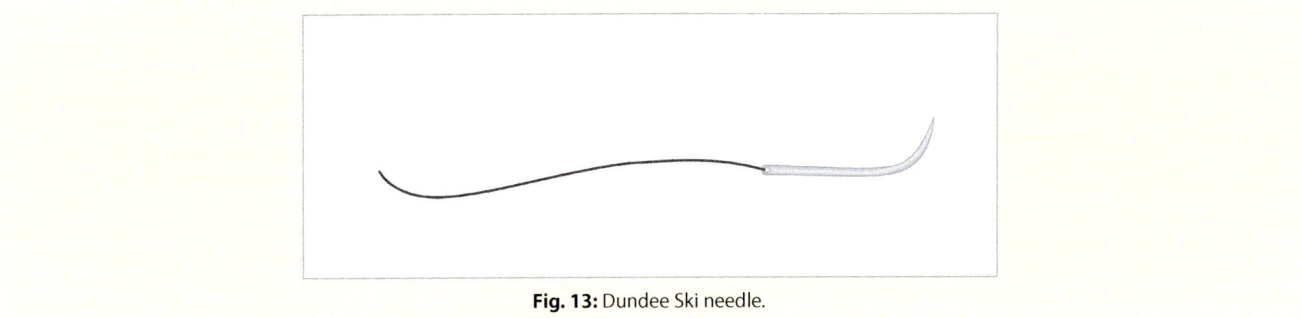

**Fig. 13:** Dundee Ski needle.

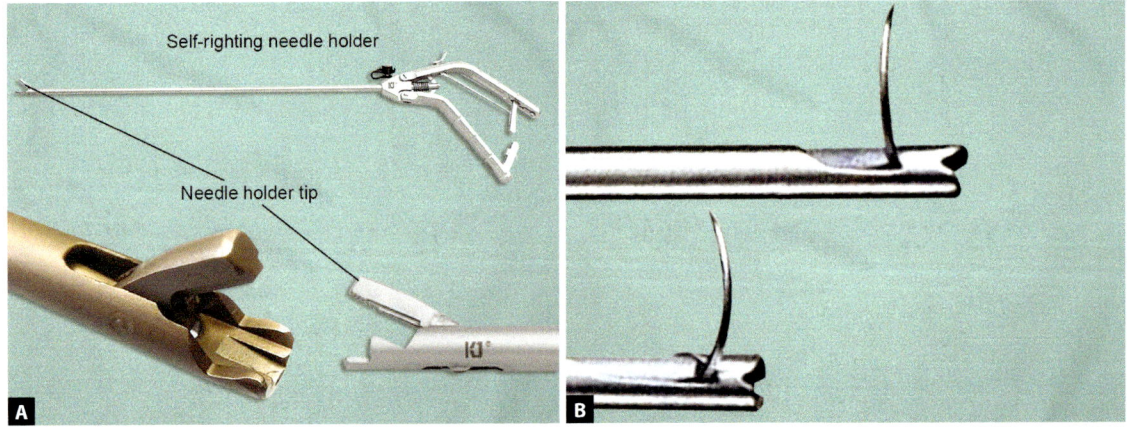

**Figs. 14A and B:** Coaxial handle laparoscopic needle holder. Coaxial type is better than pistol type, which reduces the strain with optimum maneuverability and rotation. Needle driver should be held with dominant hand; assisting instrument/grasper should be held with nondominant hand. 5-mm atraumatic grasper without ratchet is ideal.

**Figs. 15A and B:** Self-righting needle holder; it helps in positioning needle holder in-between the jaws automatically but knotting is difficult in this instrument; it can be used only for tissue penetration.

by either through "C" loop or "O" loop. *Square knot, square slip knot* **(Fig. 17)** (square knot untumbled to form slip knot), ligature slip knot, and surgeon's knot are used. Jamming slip knot and Aberdeen knot (terminal knot) are other knots, which can be placed. *Intracorporeal twist technique* is another method used in laparoscopic suturing **(Fig. 18)**. One end of the suture is rotated over the needle holder with suture tip holding for three loops; other grasper/needle holder holding other end of the suture is released to hold tip of the looped suture material; needle holder of the looped suture releases the tip of the looped suture and is allowed to hold and create a loop of the free other end of the suture, which after releasing the loop across this loop forms a knot; further pull releases the loop achieving a firm knot.

*Jamming slip knot* is a starter knot used in continuous suturing **(Figs. 19A to C)**. After double looping through needle holder, little away from the end, the suture is grasped to form a loop to which knot is slipped and further knots tighten it. This knot near the end of the suture material acts as a first knot of the continuous suture, which avoids intracorporeal knotting and hastens the suturing.

*Knot security is most important*. Here, *loosening and unraveling* of the knot should be avoided. First half knot once placed securely causes adequate tissue apposition, it should hold until second half knot is configured and cinched down on top of the first. If first half knot gets loosened (which is the holding half knot) during the formation and completion of second half

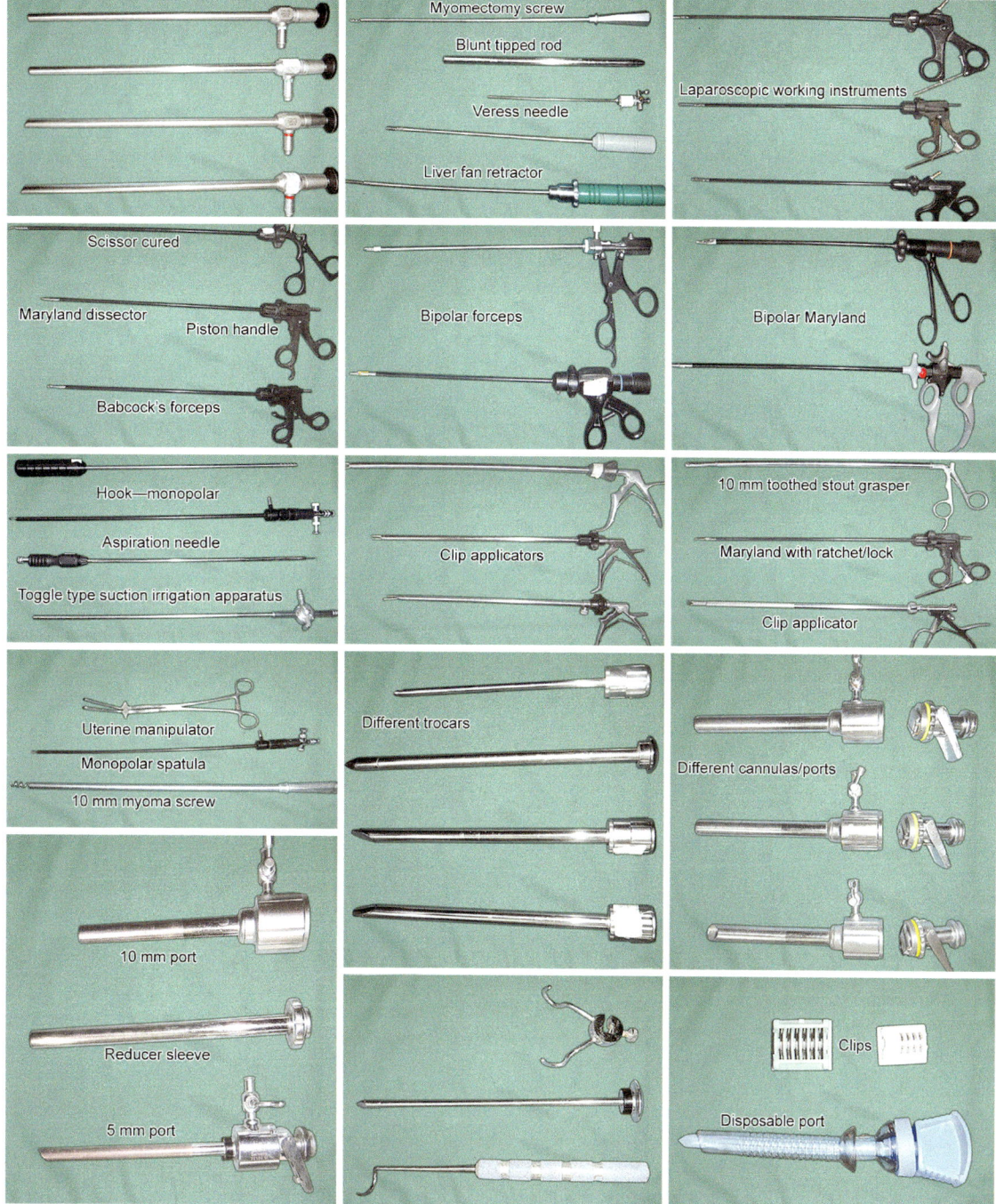

**Fig. 16:** Different laparoscopic instruments.

knot then second half knot gets locked little away from the tissue leading into improper apposition of the tissues. Braided suture material reduces the chances of first half knot slippage; surgeon's knot if placed, loosening chances reduce. *Causes for unraveling are*—cutting tail end too short, monofilament suture material with high memory (polypropylene), and lubricated or coated suture material got more chance of unraveling. While picking the knot ears, both ears should be picked up and with alignment otherwise knot unraveling and loosening is likely. It is difficult to correct an unraveled completed knot. Either knot should be cut and removed and fresh knot should be placed or one more new suture and knot is placed adjacent to unraveled knot to complete the hydrostatic suture line (seal). *Hydrostatic seal* is essential in gastrointestinal and tubular structure suturing.

*Coaxial needle holder is better.* It improves the efficiency and manipulations to achieve the proper suturing. After taking the bite through the tissue and pulling apart, part left behind prior part of the tissue bite is called as *tail end or trailing end*; part, which is on the other side and is close to the needle, is called as *standing part*; part immediately after the exit point, which is used for looping to create a knot, is called as "*bight*" (**Fig. 20**).

*Different knots can be used*—reef, surgeon's, slip, multiple, and Mayo knot. After bite of the tissue, knot should be placed and is called as *starter knot*; in continuous, sutures knot should be placed at the end and is called as *terminal knot*. It is done either by knotting to the last loop of the suture part or by Aberdeen knotting.

*First half knot* is called as flat knot/overhand knot/often hitch knot. There are two methods to achieve this mainly in laparoscopic suturing—one is by *overwrap*

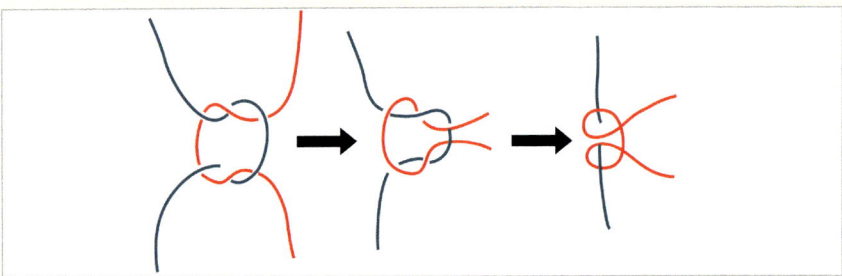

**Fig. 17:** Square knot untumbled to form slip knot—square slip knot. It has got ability to secure the knot in difficult places. It can be placed using monofilament suture material. It maintains adequate tissue tension. It is pushed in place by sliding.

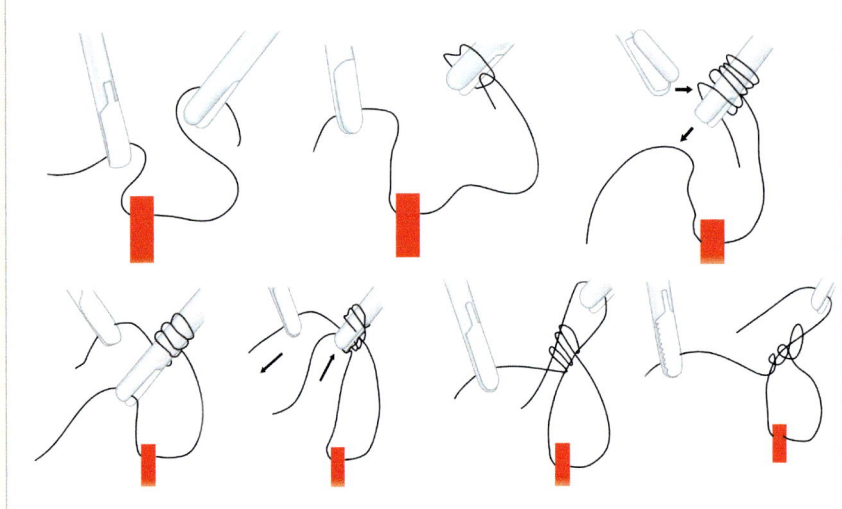

**Fig. 18:** Intracorporeal twist knotting.

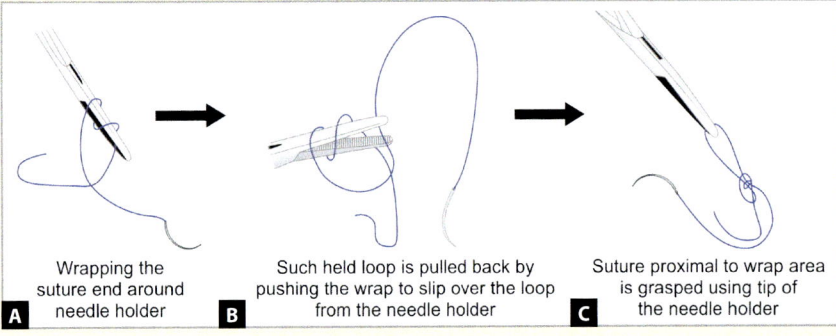

A: Wrapping the suture end around needle holder
B: Such held loop is pulled back by pushing the wrap to slip over the loop from the needle holder
C: Suture proximal to wrap area is grasped using tip of the needle holder

**Figs. 19A to C:** Jamming slip knot.

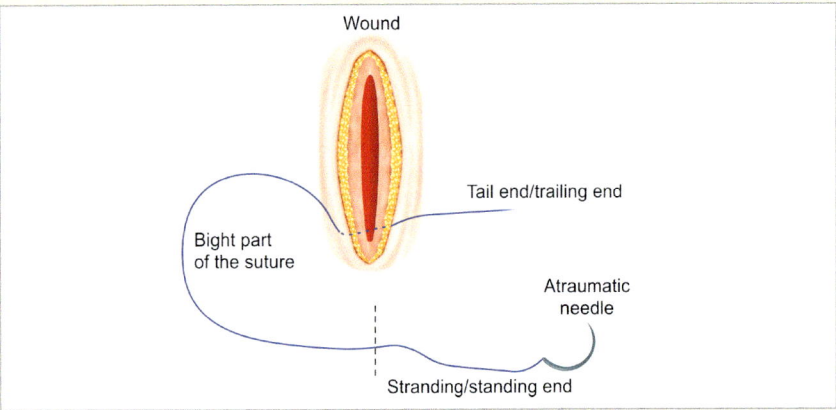

**Fig. 20:** Parts of the suture material with needle during usage after taking bite through the tissue. (1) Tail/trailing end; (2) bight where C loop is made to create knot (bight is often also called as horizon); to have proper C loop, bight should be around 2-cm length not more or not less; (3) standing (means stationary position) end/stranding end (fiber end), which is close to needle swage (both standing and stranding terminologies are used).

*method*, which is better and commonly used wherein assisting instrument is placed over the bight of the suture and is wrapped first over and then under the suture material. Here, one circle (revolution) of the bight is sufficient to achieve a half knot. Other is *underwrap method*, here assisting instrument is placed under the bight first then it is wrapped under it and over it again creating one and half circle to complete half knot. Underwrap is technically difficult. Either "C" loop or "reverse C" loop can be taken by the assisting instrument over the bight depending on the need.

### Principles in Intracorporeal Suturing and Knotting

- *Selection of proper suture gauge:* Very thin and very thick sutures are difficult to manipulate in intracorporeal knotting. Usually, 2-0 or 3-0 suture material is used. Length of the suture material should be neither too long nor too small. Usually, 10-cm length for first suture bite and additional bites require additional 2 cm for each tissue bites to complete the continuous suture of the tissues.
- *Triangulation should be optimum.* Camera port should be at the center; two working ports right and left should be on either side. Angle in which instrument enters the peritoneal cavity should be around 60°. Proper ergonomics is essential in art of laparoscopic suturing.
- *Camera of good quality with adequate magnification* is needed. Experienced camera person is important. Magnified image improves the visual perception, eye–hand coordination, and recognition of tissues. Visual image should formulate into correct judgment to configure the need. In open surgery, image is real one; in laparoscopic surgery, image is apparent, which is passed through telescope and CCD camera (charge couple device) **(Figs. 21 and 22)**.
- *Procedure steps* should be planned carefully—suturing, knotting, and so on. Slow, concentrated, smooth, and choreographic structural movement with economy of motion is essential—*Hare and hound principle*.
- *Motivation, commitment, dexterity, perfection, technical ability, and aptitude to learn* are the essential needs for laparoscopic suturing and knotting.
- *The instruments should never cross over each other* in operative field (*no crosssword principle*). Instruments should stay toward its side; if it is needed to place on opposite side, opposite side instrument should be moved laterally to avoid crossing and restriction of instrument manipulations and view too.

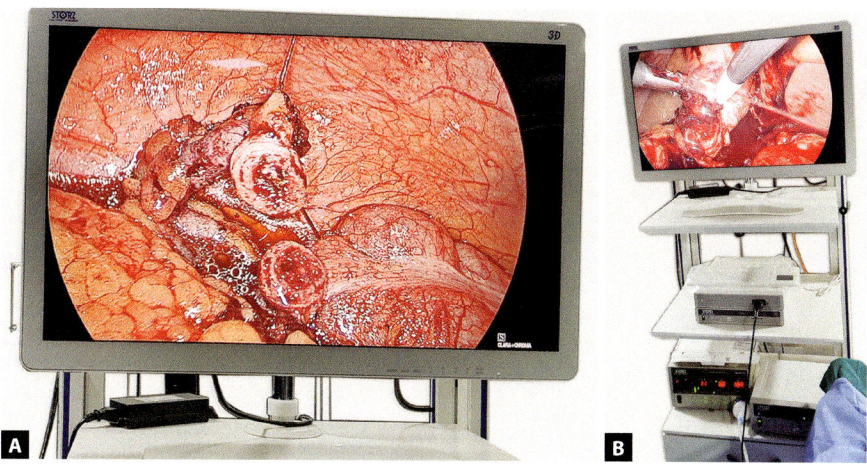

**Figs. 21A and B:** High-definition (HD) camera and monitor should be used for laparoscopic tissue approximation.

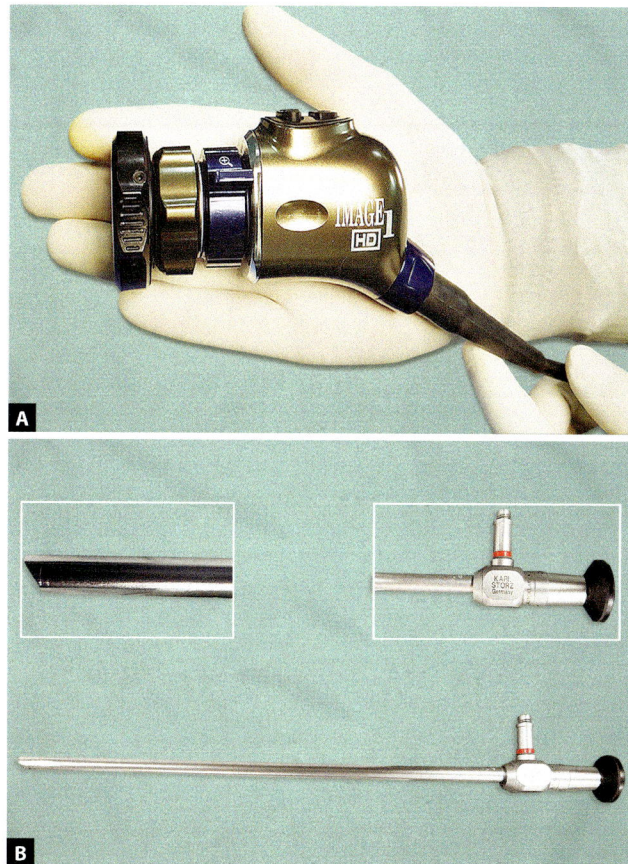

**Figs. 22A and B:** High-definition (HD) camera and 30° telescope are ideal and must for laparoscopic suturing.

- *Number of ports should be adequate.* One for camera, two as surgeon's working or suturing ports with triangulation, and additional ports as per need should be used to retract the tissues to facilitate the perfect exposure of the field. Relation of the optical port to suture line, optical alignment, proper optical viewing angle, magnification, and close-up and far viewing as per need during the technique of suturing and knotting are the essential arrangements. Angle between the two suturing instruments (45–90°) mirror image orientation (reverse alignment) and ideal direction of the movements (right side: 2–8 o'clock position; left side: 11–5 o'clock position) are important.
- *Height of the monitor* should be at the eye level of the surgeon with slightly *"gaze down"* position **(Fig. 23)**. Gaze up position will create the visual strain with recurrent neck sprain to the surgeon. Distance between the monitor and surgeon is approximately 1.5 m or 2–3 times the width of the monitor.
- *Separate monitor* is better for assistant. Surgeon and camera person usually share the same monitor for effective coordination and synchronization. *Position of the surgeon* is important; he may stand in center or on one side depending on the type of surgery and underlying anatomical relation **(Fig. 24)**.
- *Height of the table* should be at or just below the level of the elbow of the surgeon or of the tallest member of the team. More height of the table leads into poor coordination of hand movements and more fatigue and sprain. Stance of the surgeon should be optimum and comfortable. Natural position is ideal, i.e., the laparoscope is located between the right and left instruments. The offset position is used only when instrument pair is situated on one side of the laparoscope.
- *Needle driver should be parallel to the suture line.* Assisting instrument should be at 60–90° as manipulation angle. Length of the instrument is 30 cm with approximately 15 cm inside (intracorporeally). About 7–15 cm of distance from instrument tip to target tissue is good ergonomic approach.
- *Needle introduction to the abdomen cavity:* It can be done by various methods—(1) *Using 5 mm reducer*—needle holder is passed through the reducer and suture material few cm (1–2 cm) distal to the needle is grasped gently and dragged inside the reducer along with needle, so that entire suture with needle will be inside the reducer and reducer is pushed into the abdominal cavity. *Removal of the needle* is also done the same way in reverse fashion using 5-mm reducer by holding suture material 1–2 cm away from the swage end of the needle using needle holder passed across the reducer and pulled into the reducer and removed along with reducer outside; (2) *percutaneous directly*; (3) through 5-mm port by *Reich method*—here, 5-mm port is pulled out, needle holder is passed through the 5-mm port outside the abdomen, and suture is grasped close to needle and is gently passed through port wound/track along with 5-mm port into the abdominal cavity. Needle and suture entering into peritoneal cavity is visualized through the scope; (4) passing directly through 10-mm camera port after removing the telescope by holding the needle through the needle holder and advancing gently inside the peritoneal cavity; care should

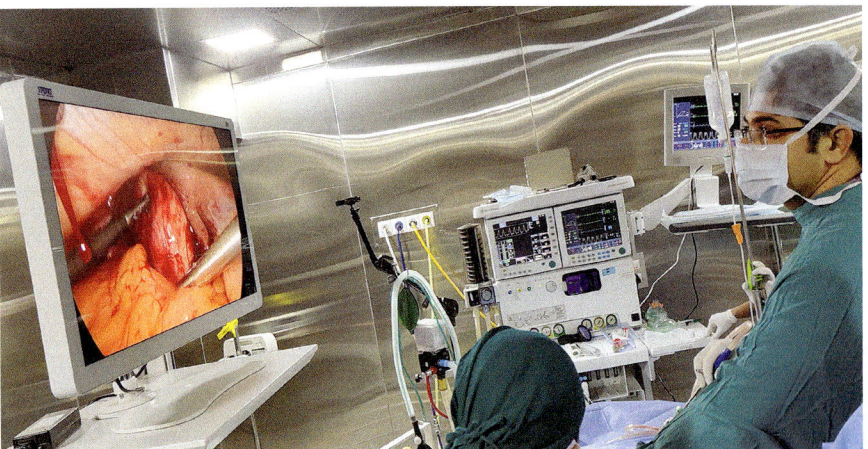

**Fig. 23:** Height of the monitor should be adjusted as "gaze down" position in laparoscopic surgery.

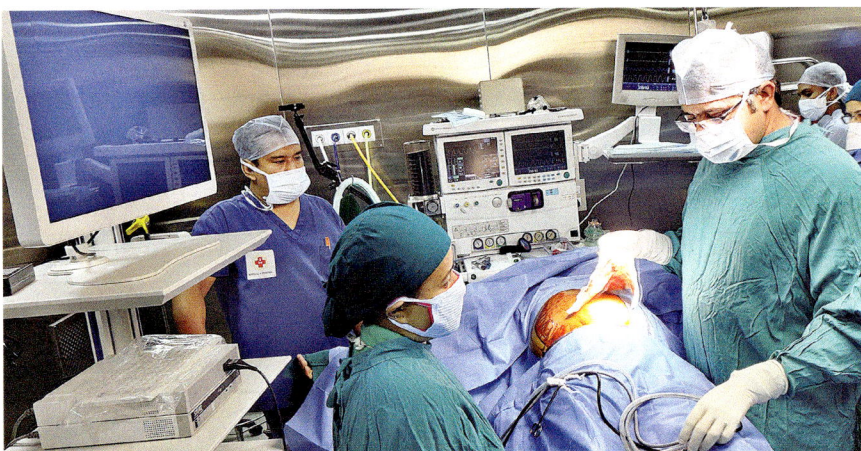

**Fig. 24:** Position, stance of the surgeon is very important in laparoscopic tissue approximation.

be taken so that direction of the port tip should be in a safer area in the peritoneal cavity to drop the needle without vision and later confirmed for place and use after passing the laparoscope through the same 10-mm camera port **(Figs. 25A to S)**.

- *Loading the needle* is often very tricky work. Suture is grasped first away (2 cm) from the swage with assisting instrument; tip of the needle is placed over a safe tissue; needle is rotated in the direction perpendicular to jaws of the needle holder; needle is grasped at the junction of proximal 1/3rd to distal 2/3rd of the jaws. Here, static part of the jaw is placed behind/beneath the needle and mobile jaw is closed over the needle with adjustment so much, so that needle erects in perpendicular position; center of the needle should be placed at the junction of the proximal 1/3rd and distal 2/3rd or as per need depending on the situation. Needle should not be held at tip. Adjusting the needle suitably needs proper maneuver, which needs concentration. *Aligning and erecting the needle carefully is essential*. Needle is locked once ideal position is confirmed. Needle is held with minimum grip while holding, but tight grip is needed while taking the tissue bite **(Figs. 26A to D)**.
- *Driving the needle across the tissue* is important. Proper *entry bite* of first edge and adequate tissue bite then proper *exit bite* of other edge with proper movements are important. *Amount of tissue bite* depends on amount of entrance and exit bites. Exit bite is easier than entrance bite in laparoscopic suturing **(Figs. 27A and B)**.
- *Knot execution:* Knot should be *executed* close to the tissue edges to be approximated to reduce the problems of depth perception. Instruments used for knotting are called as—*(1) driver instrument and (2) assisting instrument*. Driver is the one, which holds the stranding end; assisting instrument makes the needed loop to create half knot. Driver is the active instrument called as active or *dominant instrument*; instrument through which bight is looped around is called as passive or *assisting instrument*. Instrument should be kept closed (*jaw closed—mouth shut principle*). Only when needed to use to hold needle or suture jaw should be opened. *Tail end* should be of around 1.5 cm in length, so that knotting will be easier and further bites and *terminal knots* will be better, as suture is saved and also avoids extra work of removing the suture piece and passing additional suture material intracorporeally—*Canny Scot principle*. This avoids needle loss too.
- *Directional suture hold:* Assisting instrument to make C loop should be on the side where tail is present; *right is right, left is left*. For example, if tail is on the right side, standing part is held with left instrument and C loop is created with right side instrument to complete *the first half knot*; second half knot is completed by changing the method, i.e., right instrument will hold the standing end and left instrument creates the C loop.
- *Bight size should optimum* and should not be too small or should not be too long; if it is too small, tail may slip off the tissue or creation of C loop will be difficult; if bight is too long then sliding down the loop will be difficult by entanglement and may form S loop.
- *Overwrapping is better* always while creating half knot. Proper choreography is important. *Wrapping is always superior than twirling the instrument*; to a beginner twirling the instrument looks easier but *wrapping the bight is the ideal method. Steps needed are*—(1) orienting the bight to create proper shape; (2) holding the thread; and (3) making torque to create loop. Bight must lie evenly. Suture material should be held proximal to bight area; circular needle should not be held while creating the loop (endoski needle can be grasped) unless bight part has become too small to create half moon. Angle between the two instruments should be around 40–60°. After wrapping, jaw of the assisting instrument is advanced toward the tail of the suture material to pick up; once picked up, jaws should close firmly to avoid slippage of the held suture material and wrapped suture is spilled over the tail of the suture to create firm half knot; it should *be cinched properly* to achieve optimum tissue approximation. Squaring should be done at this point. Second half knot is created again using opposite instruments, as tail end stays now on the contralateral side. Tail is held with assisting instrument while tightening the knot with active instrument giving distraction force **(Figs. 28A to C)**.

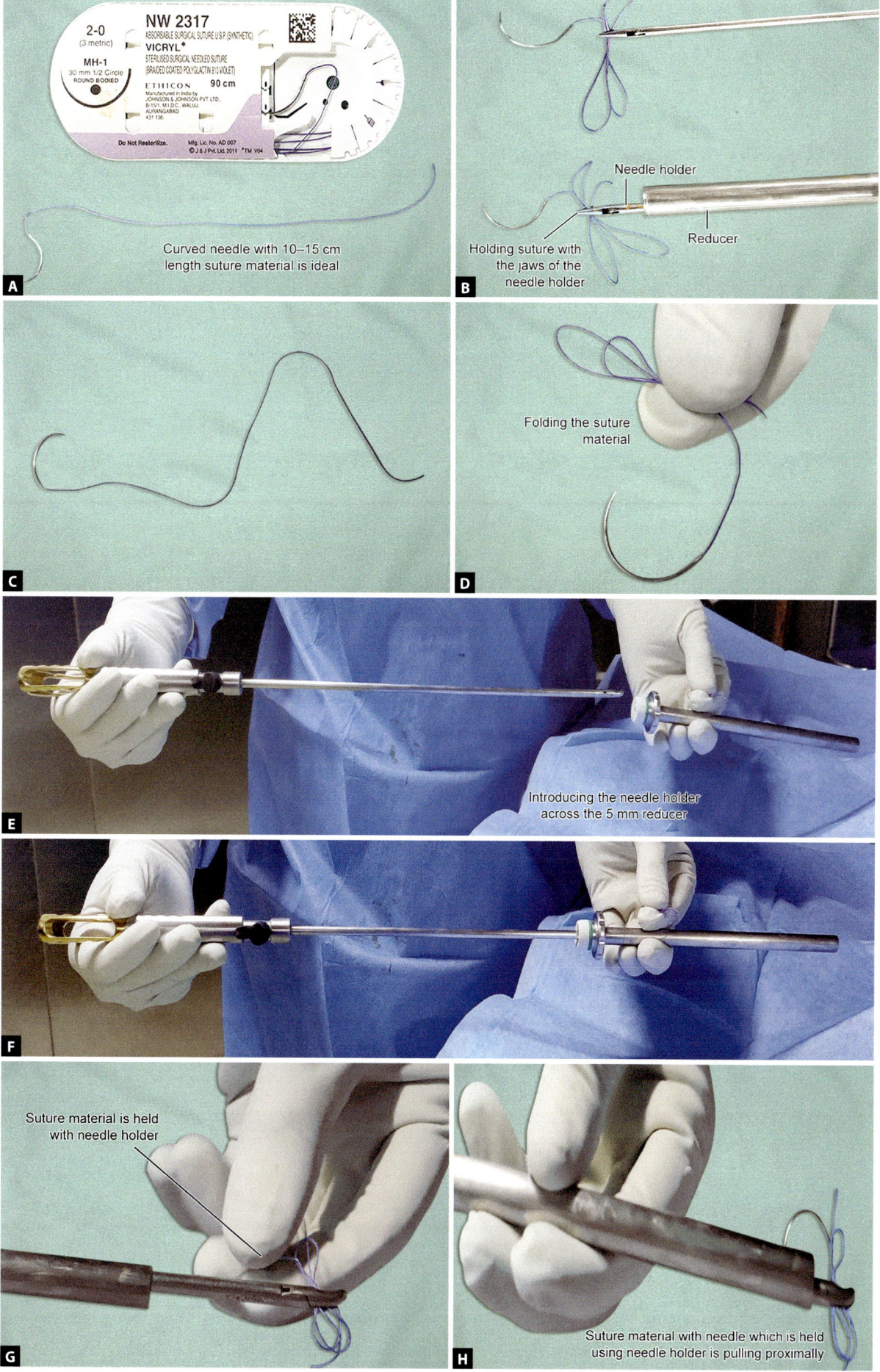

Figs. 25A to H

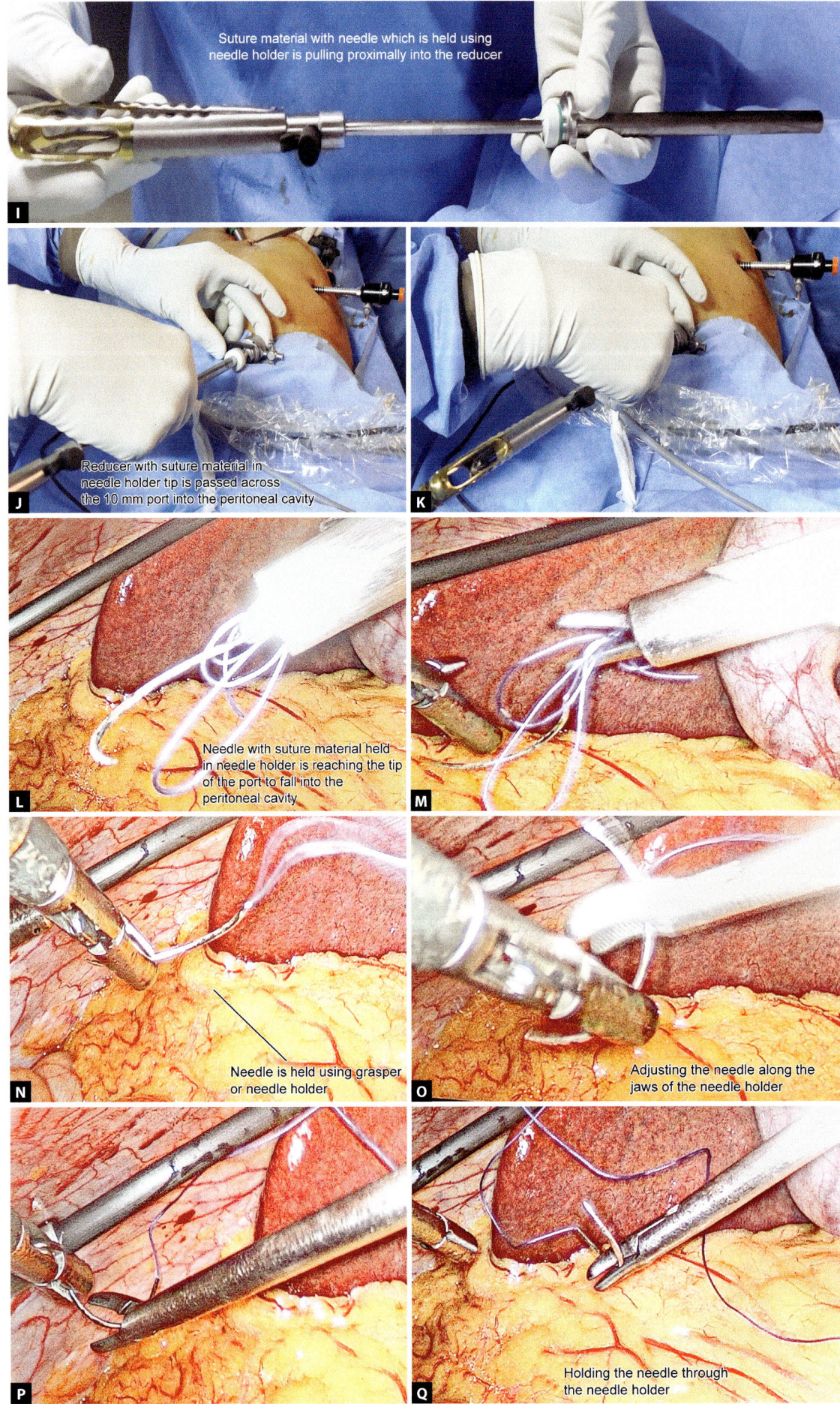

Figs. 25I to Q

Laparoscopic Suturing and Knotting

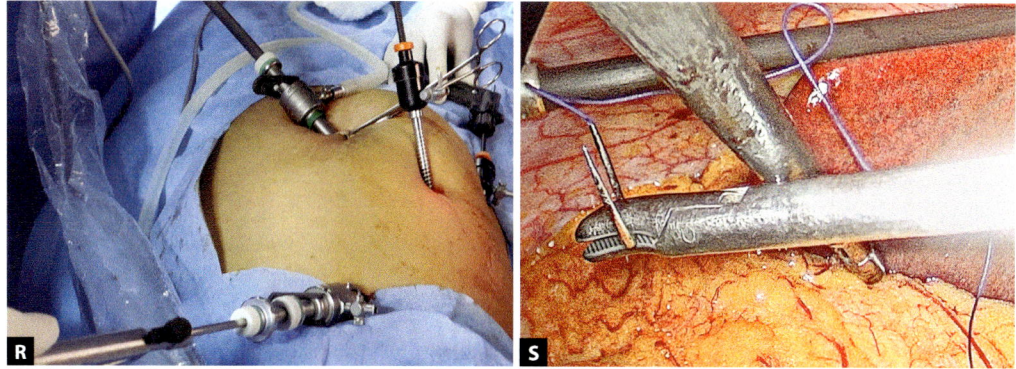

**Figs. 25R and S**

**Figs. 25A to S:** Method of introduction of the needle with suture material into the peritoneal cavity—standard method through 10-mm working port using 5-mm reducer.

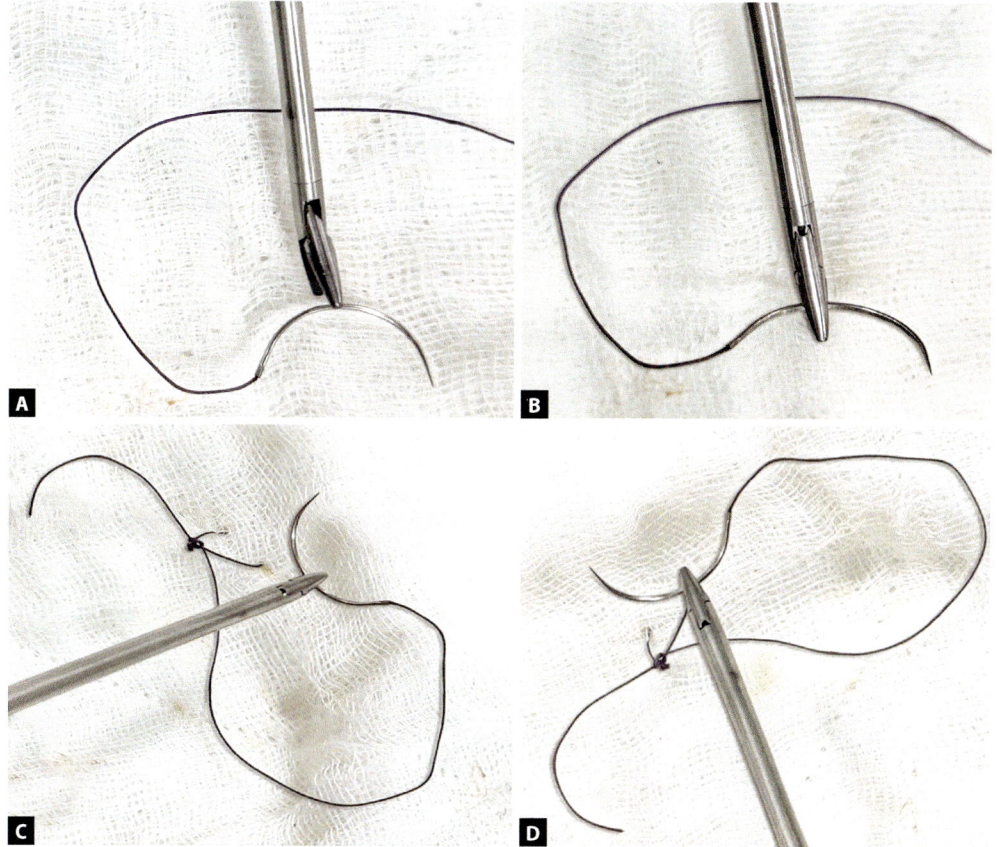

**Figs. 26A to D:** Holding, erecting, and aligning the needle into the needle holder.

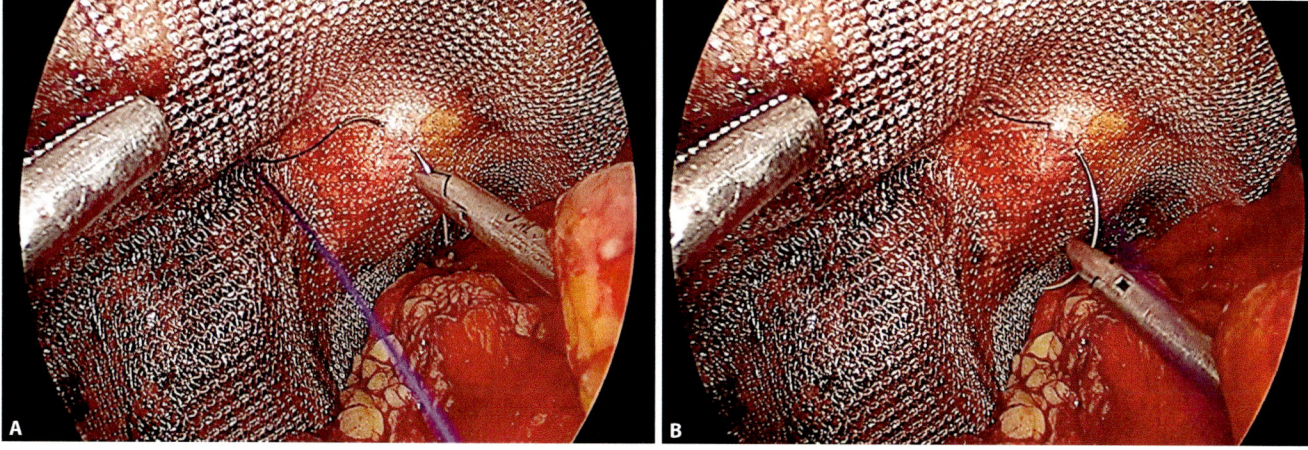

**Figs. 27A and B:** Laparoscopic suturing—taking tissue bites in intracorporeal suturing.
*Courtesy:* Dr Ganesh MK, Laparoscopic Surgeon, Father Muller's Hospital and Medical College, Mangaluru, Karnataka

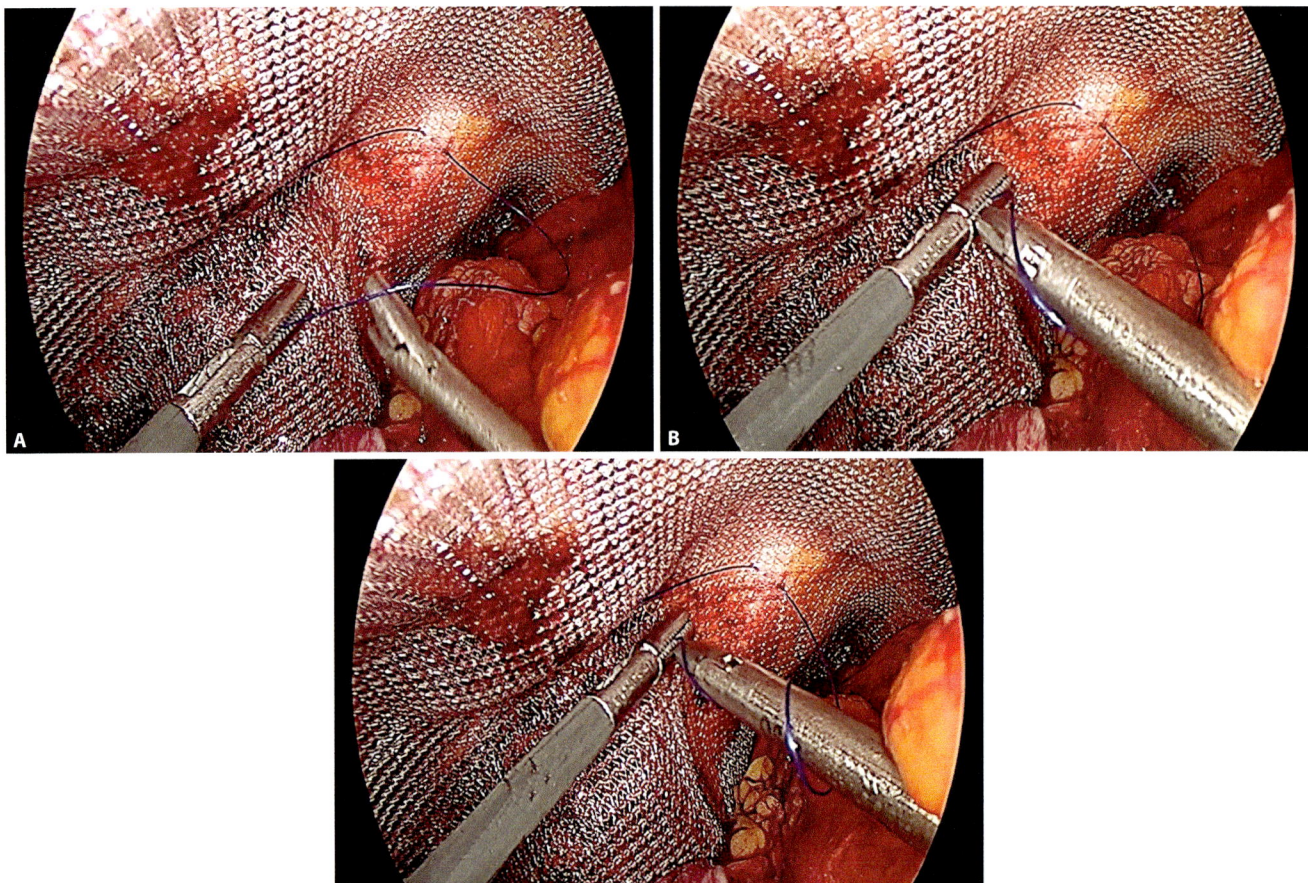

**Figs. 28A to C:** Instrument knotting in laparoscopic surgery (intracorporeal knotting).
*Courtesy:* Dr Ganesh MK; Laparoscopic Surgeon, Father Muller's Hospital and Medical College, Mangaluru, Karnataka

- *Hand movements* should have enhanced level of coordinated ambidexterity and with both hands should work equally and precisely. Finger, wrist, forearm supination, and pronation should be coordinated properly. Visual perception should lead into judgment and planning and thereby execution through both hands. Productive economy movements with avoidance of unnecessary movements (*flawless technique*) to prevent errors which lead slow steady perfect execution.

- *Outcome and quality of tissue approximation* should be equivalent to open technique without any compromise. Right technique with performance standards should be called for **(Figs. 29A to P)**.

*Sequence of events in laparoscopic tissue approximation:*
Selection of the suture material, size, and needle → selection of the proper length of the suture material → passing the needle with suture material into the peritoneal cavity → loading the needle into needle driver → adjusting the needle → handling the needle and driving the needle through entrance and exit bites of the tissue → orientation for the proper knot execution → keeping the tail end optimum 1.5–2 cm only → holding the stranding end using driving instrument (right is right, left is left) → assisting instrument creates C loop through bight part of the suture material → through assisting instrument, tail end of the suture material is held and firmly locked → loop is spilled over the jaws into the tail → half knot squared and cinched firmly on to the tissue to avoid slipping or unraveling → second half knot is placed using opposite hands this time and suture strand should be kept loose to avoid unraveling.

## REMEMBER

### Suturing
- Repetitive self-learning is essential to master intracorporeal suturing and knotting.
- Needle holder/driver should be parallel to suture line.
- Needle should be in perpendicular position to the suture line.
- Needle should be grasped tightly while taking tissue bite.
- There should be proper triangulation and visibility of both instruments
- No cross-sword phenomenon during manipulation **(Fig. 30)**.
- Proper thick entrance and exit tissue bites should be taken.
- Needle should not be held at the tip.

### Knotting
*Two methods are available:* (1) "C" loop method, which is commonly used and (2) "Gladiator Rule" method.
- "C" loop method:
  - For first half knot, right-hand instrument is driving instrument and left-hand instrument is assisting instrument.
  - Standing end is held with right-hand driving instrument and suture material is looped (overwrap) on the stationary left-hand instrument along the bight (horizon); second loop (double loop) can be taken to make surgeon's knot.

*Contd...*

## Laparoscopic Suturing and Knotting

*Contd...*

- Both instruments gently moved toward the tail end (1.5–2 cm length) and jaws of left-hand assisting instrument, which is having looped suture, are opened to grasp the tail end and held firmly.
- Loop is gently spilled over the tail and cinched and first half knot is created by pulling the instruments opposite direction.
- Second half knot is done through opposite hands (here now right hand will become assisting and left hand becomes driving instruments) and loop is created from behind to achieve square knot (reef).
- Additional third half knot is placed to secure further wherein loop is done as alike first half knot.

- *"Gladiator Rule" method:* Here, assisting instrument holds the suture material 2 cm proximal to create *horizon or bight*; needle holder with open jaw passes first in front of the horizon then behind it by rotating the needle holder 180° around its axis; needle holder further moves behind the suture (horizon/bight) to rotate further 180° to come back to its original position; additional turn can be created similarly to have surgeon's knot (double half knot); needle holder grasps the tail of the suture material and is pulled in opposite direction to create *first half knot*.

    *Second half knot* is created same way with same needle holder rotating around the bight/horizon of the suture material but first from behind to create a second "reverse half knot"; by pulling in opposite direction, squaring is done.

    *Third half knot* is created to support initial two half knots, which is done same way as first half knot using needle holder to loop the bight part of the suture material.

    "Gladiator rule" is similar to open instrument knotting method, so surgeons often prefer this method but "C" loop method is more secure.

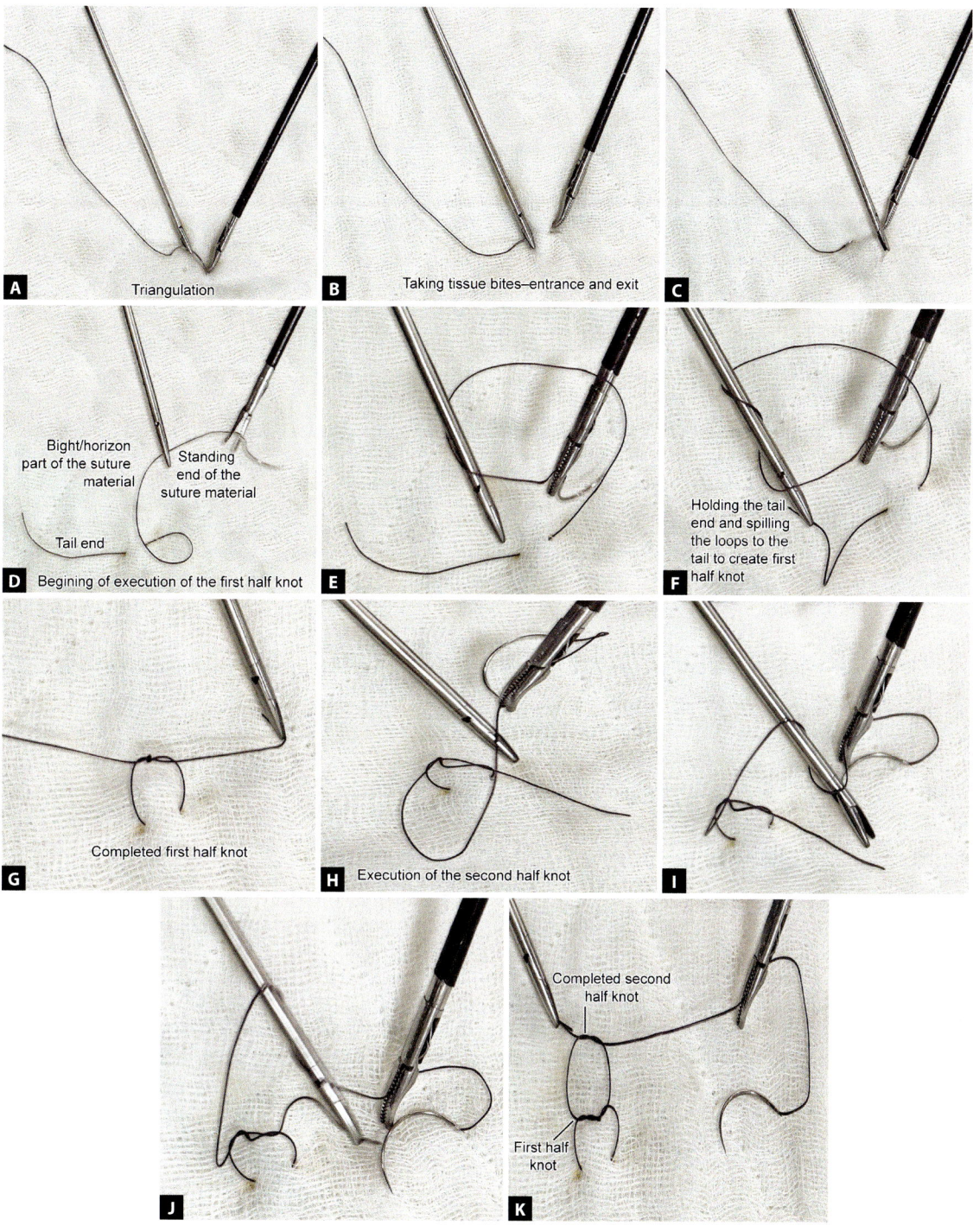

**Figs. 29A to K**

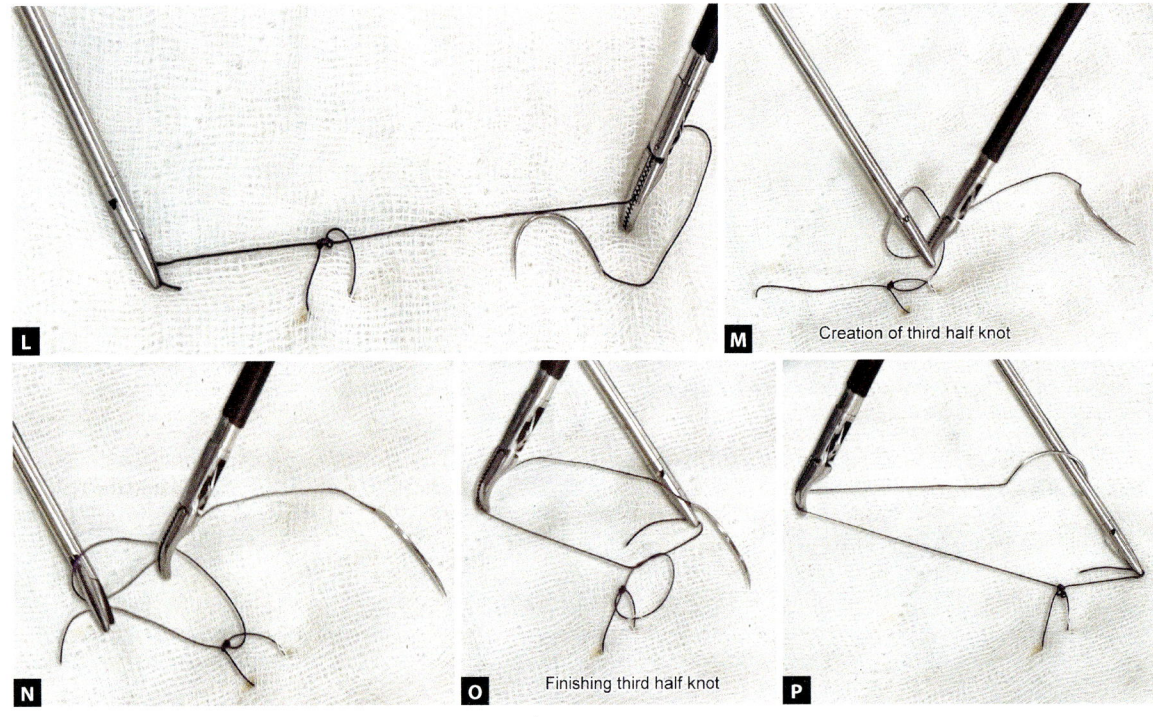

**Figs. 29L to P**

**Figs. 29A to P:** Intracorporeal suturing technique (demonstration); note the execution of first, second, and third half knots.
*Courtesy:* Dr Keshvaprasad, Associate Professor, Laparoscopic Surgeon, KMC, Mangaluru, Karnataka

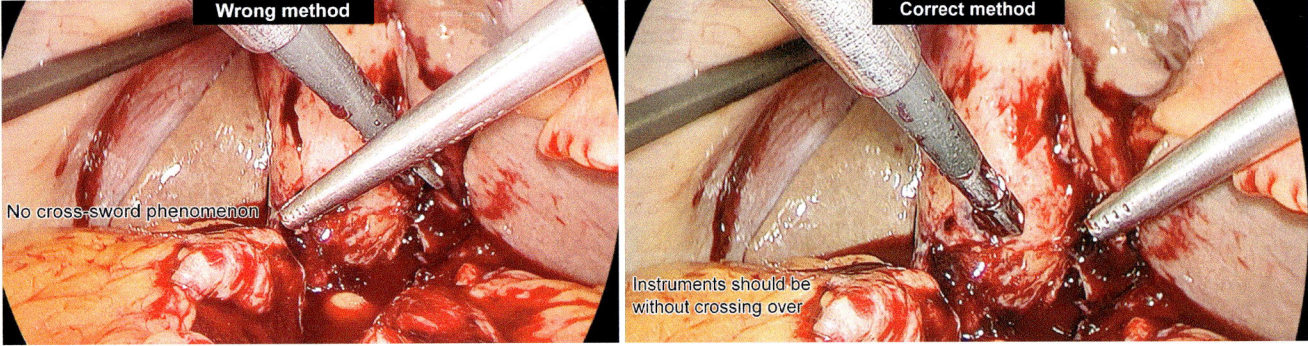

**Fig. 30:** During laparoscopic surgery, instruments should not crossover—no cross-sword phenomenon.

## PROBLEMS AND ERRORS IN LAPAROSCOPIC TISSUE APPROXIMATION

- *Loosening of the knot:* It is commonly seen while tying the first half knot. It is due to lack of technical skill, tissue friability, and suture material type (if monofilament). It can be overcome by proper tightening the first half knot, careful spilling over the second half knot later, and tightening the second half knot firmly. Third half knot will give additional security.
- *Short suture length:* In order to make manipulation easier, short length of the suture is used and often it becomes inadequate length to finish the suturing, and terminal knot placement becomes difficult. It can be done by making *half-moon effect* on the suture or by holding the needle with needle holder **(Fig. 31)**.

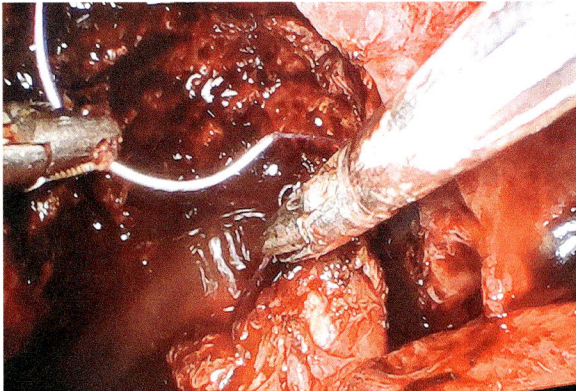

**Fig. 31:** Half-moon needle technique is used when difficulty arises for creating the knot due to short bight.

- *Creation of wrong loop:* Formation of "S" loop or "Reverse S" loop by holding the suture with wrong hand can occur or knot tying above the stitch creating "O" loop—all these will lead into incorrect unsafe knot (flat knot cannot be created by this).
- *Unraveling of knot:* It is due to improper method, or slippery suture material. At the end, if the knot requires to be

held, it should be done by holding both ears (tails) of the knot otherwise (if one ear is held) knot will unravel. It is better not to touch unraveled knot; safer is to place one more suture and knot in close proximity to this knot.

- *Instrument crossing creating cross-sword problems* makes manipulation difficult or impossible.
- *Needle deflection can occur*, making needle to pass through at different place than actual plan. It needs proper but soft grip and precise firm dedicated movement of the needle.
- *Missing the needle or breaking of the needle tip* may be a problem. This is often very difficult to manage, as needle may get lost anywhere in the abdomen or pelvis or interloop and so on. C-arm radiological localization and use of the magnetized probe may be helpful. Laparotomy and localization may be needed in few situations.
- *Injury to major vessels by improper direction* of the needle during movement will cause prick on the vessels. It often may lead into torrential bleeding. Remove the needle from the vessel gently and carefully; apply pressure after placing the radiopaque gauze into the field through 10-mm port using 5-mm reducer. Firm pressure on the site usually stops the bleeding. It can be prevented by keeping the needle continuously under view and avoiding the holding of the needle unnecessarily other than during suturing.

## RETRIEVAL OF THE NEEDLE WITH SUTURE MATERIAL

After placing suture and knot in laparoscopic surgery (intracorporeal suturing), safe removal of the needle with suture is very important. As often suture material attached to the needle becomes small in length after execution of the suturing, there is chances of needle getting missed may cause real trouble to retrieve it outside. Needle should be placed in safe place either over a solid organ or on the abdominal wall. Through 10 mm port reducer with needle holder is passed into the peritoneal cavity. Remaining thread part in the needle (not directly on the needle) is held firmly using needle holder. Proper firm grasping is important. Camera should be focused on the needle and needle holder and focusing should be followed while moving the held needle towards the reducer proximally. Care should be taken so that needle will not fall into the peritoneal cavity inadvertently. Entire event is observed until the entire needle disappears into the reducer properly. Reducer with firm grip on the needle holder is removed outside; and outside needle holder is pushed forward again across the reducer to see the tip of the needle holder with needle which is retrieved by unlocking the needle holder **(Figs. 32A to N)**.

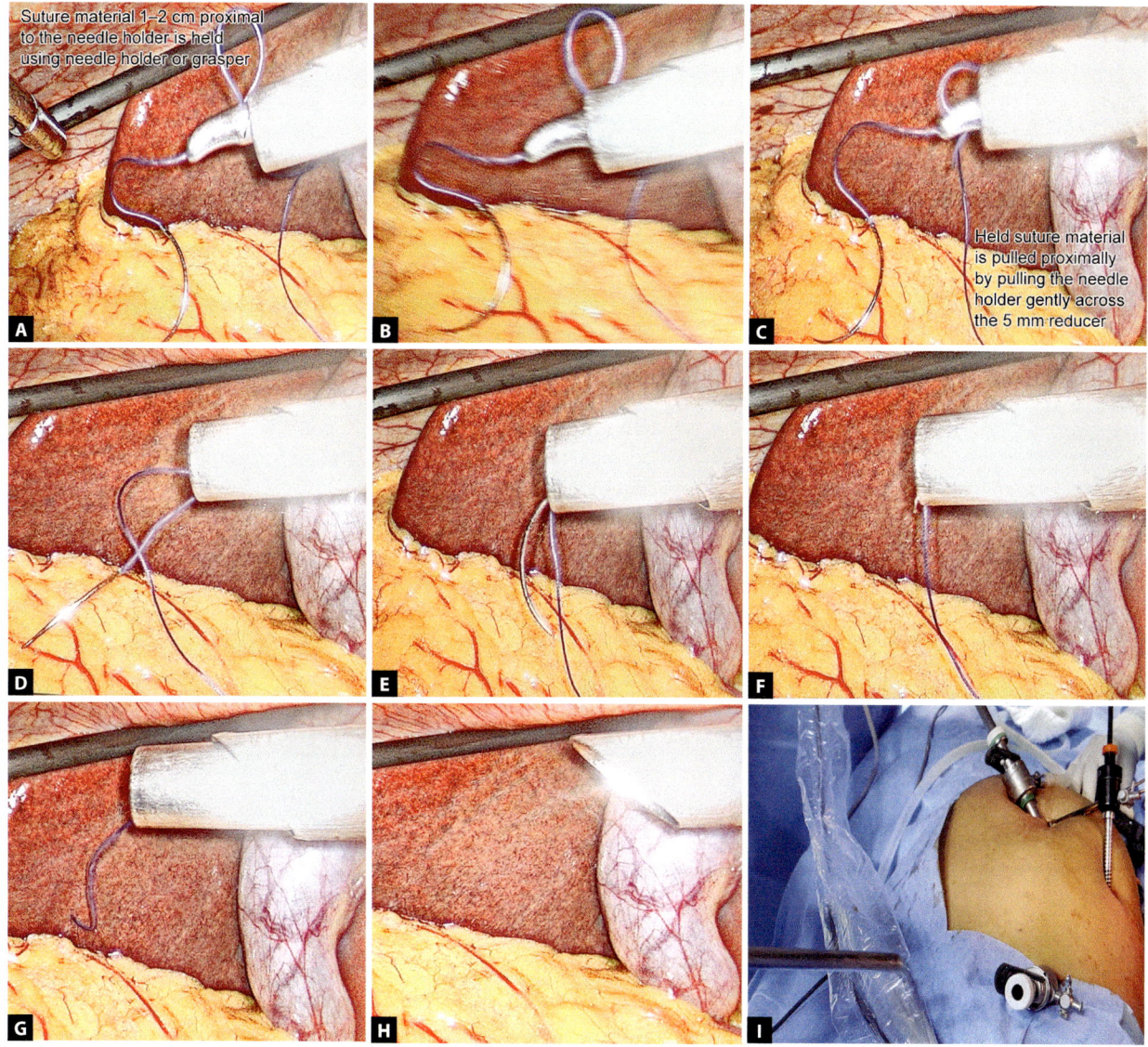

Figs. 32A to I

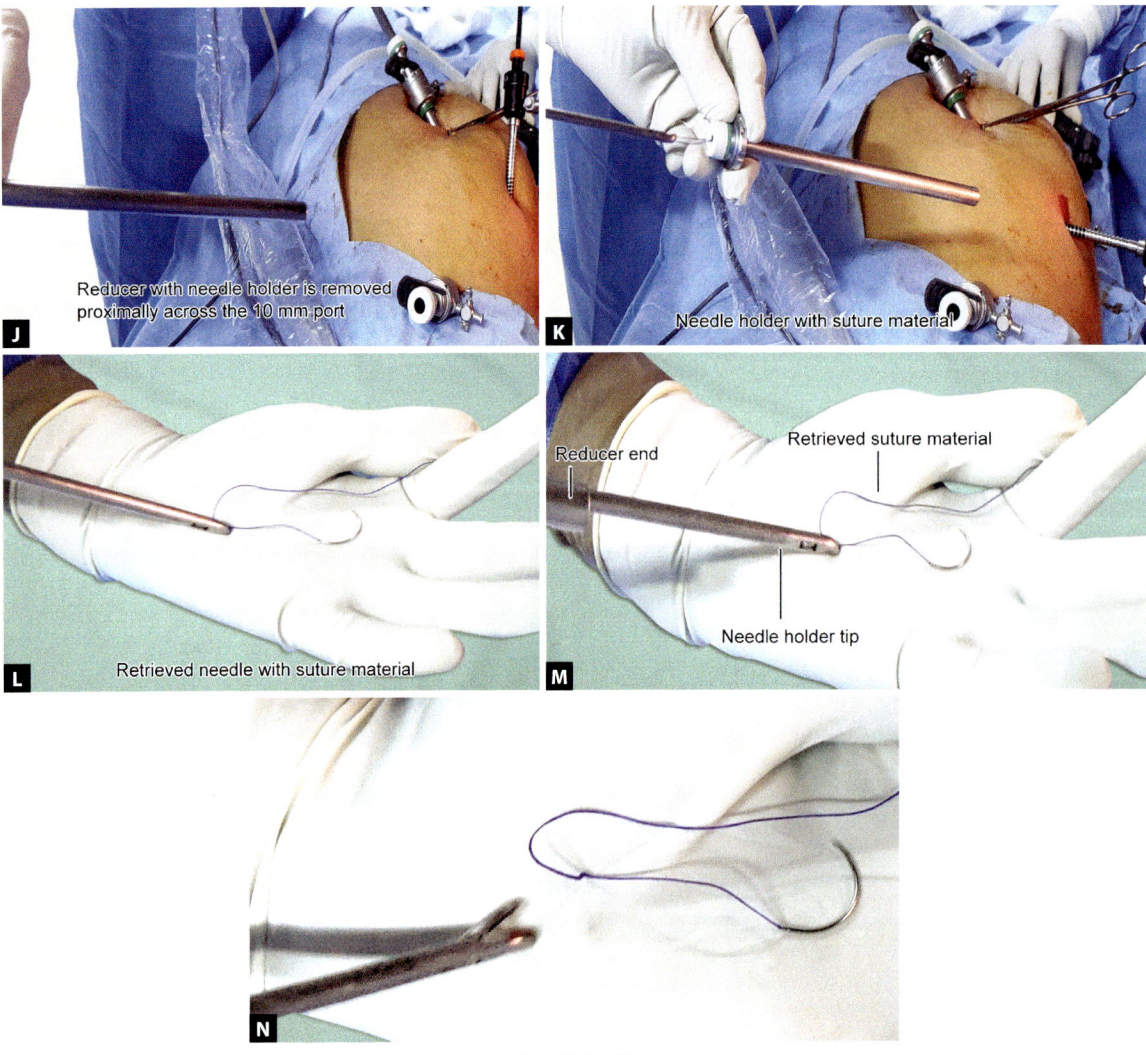

**Figs. 32J to N**

**Figs. 32A to N:** Technique of safe retrieval of the needle holder from peritoneal cavity after laparoscopic intracorporeal suturing.

# Index

## A

Aberdeen hand knot 40, 42
Absorbable suture materials 13, 16
Absorbable suture, natural 16
Absorbable suture, synthetic 16
Absorption of suture materials 15, 16
Absorption time 15
Adson's forceps 4, 6
Allgower technique 50
Ambroise Pare 1
Atraumatic needle 25

## B

BP handle 7
Barbed suture 19
Bard Parker's handle 7
Baumgartner needle holder 4, 5
Bayonet forceps 9
Bight 77, 78
Bioadhesives 12
Biology of suture materials 15
Bishop Harmon forceps 4, 6, 7
Bonney Reverdin needle 26
Breaking strength retention 15
Brown and sharpe-gauge system 19
Bunnel needle 25

## C

Capillarity 15
Catgut 1, 16
Cautery 9
Chain stitch knot 40
Classification of the surgical needle 20
Claudius Galen 1
Clip removal 9
"C" loop 78
Coaxial needle holder 73, 76, 77
Compound needles 25
Connell suture 68
Continuous "mass closure" 49
Continuous blanket sutures 49
Continuous locking suture 54
Continuous locking suture with Aberdeen knot 54
Continuous locking sutures 49
Continuous mass closure 54
Continuous over and over simple suture 49
Continuous suturing 67
Conventional cutting needle 24
Cotton 18
Crimping 22
Crooked Pare needle 21
Cross-sword, No, principle 78, 86
Curved needle 25
Cushing suture 68
Cuticular needles 25

## D

Dacron and Terylene/Polyesters 18
Diamond knives 8
Different knot tying techniques 36
Different parts of the needle 22
Different techniques to attach the needle to suture material in atraumatic eyeless needle 22
Dissecting forceps 4, 5, 7
Dog ear 42
Dolphin needle 25
Donati suture 49
Duncan slip knot 70, 72
Dundee Ski needle 76

## E

Elasticity of the suture material 15
Endoloop 71, 73
Endoloop used in ligating tubular structures 71
Endoski needle 25
Eureka needle 20, 21
Expanded polytetrafluoroethylene 19
Extracorporeal knots 73
Extracorporeal knotting 70

## F

Far-far and near-near suture 49, 50
Far-near and near-far modified vertical mattress suture 50
Features of ideal suture material 13
Features of surgical needle 21
Figure of eight suture 64
Finger tip pressure 3
Fluid movement of the wrist 28
Fundamental basis of suturing 2

## G

Galen 1
Gallie's needle 26
Gambee single layer full thickness 67
Gauze 7
George Merson 2
"Gladiator Rule" method 84, 85
Glycomer-631 16
Goals of suturing 46
Goals of the wound closure 28
Gore-Tex 19

## H

Hagedorn reverse flattened point fishhook needle 26
Half knot 2, 77
Half-moon needle 86
Halsted 2
Halsted mosquito forceps 8
Halsted suture 68
Hand knot typing 36
Haneke-Marini suture 51
Hare and Hound Principle 78
Hemostat 8
Hemostatic figure of eight suture 61
History of suturing 1
Holding the instrument 3
Holding the needle holder 3, 5, 29
Horizon 78
Horizontal mattress suture 51, 63

## I

Instrument knot tying 40
Instruments for suturing 3
Integral flanged needle 20, 21
Interrupted cruciate suture 62, 65
Interrupted suture 67
Intracorporeal knotting 84
Intracorporeal suturing and knotting 73
Intracorporeal suturing technique 86
Intracorporeal twist technique 76
Inverting horizontal mattress suture 56, 63

## J

Jamming slip knot 76, 78
JB needle 25
Jenkin's rule 32, 49
John Hunter 2
Joseph Lister 2
Juergen-Breunner needle 25

## K

Keith needle 25
Kilner needle holder 28
Knot 35
Knot components 35
Knot execution 80
Knot pusher 70
Knot tying, hand knot 36
Knot tying, instrument 40
Knot tying, stages 36
Knot, Aberdeen hand knot 40, 42
Knot, components 37
Knot, decorative 35
Knot, Duncan slip 70, 72
Knot, end 35
Knot, granny 36, 38
Knot, half 41, 77
Knot, Jamming slip 76, 78
Knot, Melzer 70, 72
Knot, modified Fisherman's 36
Knot, reef 36-38
Knot, Roeder's 70-72
Knot, self locking suture 36, 38
Knot, sheet bend 36
Knot, single hand technique 39
Knot, squaring 36
Knot, starter 35, 77
Knot, surgeon's 36, 38
Knot, sutured, components 35
Knot, Tayside 70, 72
Knot, terminal 35, 77
Knot, Texas Endosurgery Institute 70
Knot, triple modified reef 36
Knot, two-hands technique 39
Knot, utility 35
Knot-pull tensile strength 15
Kousnetzoff aluminum needle 26

## L

Lactomer copolymer 17
Lane's needle 26

Laparoscopic instruments 77
Laparoscopic needle holder 12
Laparoscopic suturing 83
Laparoscopic suturing and knotting, types 70
LE Hughes double near and far suture 67
Lembert suture 67, 68
Ligature 33
Linen 18
Loading the needle 80
Locking horizontal mattress suture 56, 63
Locking vertical mattress suture 59
Loop mattress suture 50
Loop vertical mattress locking suture 50
Loop vertical mattress suture 58

## M

Maxon 16
Mayo Hager needle holder 4, 28
Mayo needle 26
Meigster clamp 33
Melzer's knot 70, 72
Melzer's knot pusher 70
Memory of suture material 41
Mersutures 2
Micropoint needle 24
Mixter clamp 33
Modified Smead–Jones closure 66, 67
Monofilament sutures 13
Mounted tie 33
Multifilament suture 13

## N

Natural suture materials 13
Near and near; far and far vertical mattress suture (short hand) 56, 57
Near-near far-far vertical mattress suturing 50
Needle "ski" 73
Needle arming 28
Needle bite 2
Needle body 23
Needle driver 4
Needle eye 21
Needle eye types and shapes 22
Needle holder 3, 4
Needle holder, pistol 73, 76
Needle holder, coaxial 73, 76, 77
Needle holder, parts 4
Needle holder, self-righting 73, 76
Needle integrity 21
Needle length 21
Needle shoulder 23
Needle size 21
Needle surgical, ideal features of 24
Needle tapering 24
Needle tip 23
Needle types 24
Needle yield 20
Needle, diameter 21
Needle, different parts 22
Needle, radius 21
Needle, surgical, parts 21
No cross-sword principle 78, 86
Non-absorbable suture materials 13, 17
Nonabsorbable sutures 13
Nonsticky bipolar cautery 10
Non-woven gauze 7
Nylon 18

## O

Overwrap method 77, 78, 80

## P

Parts of a surgical instrument 3
Parts of a surgical needle 21
Percutaneous vertical mattress suture 51
Petit eyeless concept of a needle 21
Pistol needle holder 73, 76
Plasticity 15
Poliglecaprone-25 16
Polybutester–Novafil 19
Polydioxanone suture material 17
Polyethylene 19
Polyglactin-910 17
Polyglyconate 16
Polyglytone-621 16
Polypropylene 18
Polyvinylidene fluoride 19
Port closure needle 25
Prerequisites for laparoscopic suturing 70
Principles in Intracorporeal Suturing and Knotting 78
Principles of Knot Tying 35
Principles of Suturing 28, 32
Problems and errors in laparoscopic tissue approximation 86
Problems with laparoscopic suturing 69
Properties of the suture material 14
Pulley suture 50
Purse-string suture 62, 65

## Q

Quilled suture 65

## R

Railroad scar 15
Reich method 74, 79
Removal of the suture 32
Retention sutures 65, 66
Retrieval of the needle with suture material 87, 88
Reverse cutting needle 24
"Reverse C" loop 78
Reverse slipping 70
Rhazes of Arabia 2
Roeder's knot 70-72
Round body needle 24
Rule, Jenkin's 32, 49
Running locked suturing 48
Running vertical mattress suture 51

## S

Scalpel handle and blade 7
Scissors 8
Sectorization 69
Selection of the suture material 19
Self-righting needle holder 73, 76
Sequence of events in laparoscopic tissue approximation 84
Sergeant instrument 65
Short hand vertical mattress 50
Shuttle needle 26
Silk 17
Simple everting suture 47
Simple interrupted fascial suture 47
Simple interrupted suture placement 30, 32
Simple interrupted suturing 46
Simple running suturing 47
Single layer seromucosal suture of bowel 67
"Ski" needle 25, 73
Skin and soft tissue suturing 46
Skin stapler 9, 10
Sliming 16
Smead–Jones sutures, modified 65-67
Spatulated side cutting needle 24
Stainless steel 19
Starter knot 77
Subcuticular suture 56
Subcuticular suture placing 64
Surgical instrument, parts of 3
Surgical needles 20
Surgical slip knots 16
Sutura 1
Suture 1
Suture material classification 19
Suture materials and needles 13
Suture removal 45
Suture removal set 9
Suture tensile strength 15
Suturing, fundamental basis of 2
Swaging 22, 25
Symonds round bodied fishhook needles 26
Synthetic absorbable sutures 16

## T

Taper cut needle 24
Taper round needle 24
Tayside knot 70, 72
Technical Basis of Suturing 2
Ten Commandments in Suturing 46
Tensile strength 15
Tension suture 65, 66
Terminal knot 77
Texas Endosurgery Institute Knot 70
Three-point suture 62, 64
Throw 2
Tissue forceps 4, 5, 7
Transfixation ligature 34
Traumatic needle 26
Triangulation 69, 78
Trocar needle 25
Tru taper needle 25
Types of laparoscopic suturing and knotting 70

## U

Under wrap method 78, 80
Under-running of the tissue 34

## V

Vertical mattress pulley suture 59, 61
Vertical mattress suture 49
Vertical mattress—Allgöwer suture technique 58
Victor Bonney's toothed forceps 6
Vise like grip 3
Visiblack needle 25

## W

William Stewart Halsted 2
Wound breaking strength 15

## Y

Yasargil micro needle holder 28